AF806364

Malignant Mesothelioma and Pseudomyxoma

Mikhail V. Kiselevskiy • Amir G. Abdulaev
Mikhail M. Davydov
Editors

Malignant Mesothelioma and Pseudomyxoma

Springer

Editors
Mikhail V. Kiselevskiy
Laboratory of Cell Immunity
N.N. Blokhin National Medical
Research Center
Moscow, Russia

Mikhail M. Davydov
Oncologist and Surgeon Thoracic
Research Department
N.N. Blokhin National Medical
Research Center
Moscow, Russia

Amir G. Abdulaev
Oncologist and Surgeon Thoracic
Research Department
N.N. Blokhin National Medical
Research Center
Moscow, Russia

ISBN 978-3-319-99509-0 ISBN 978-3-319-99510-6 (eBook)
https://doi.org/10.1007/978-3-319-99510-6

Library of Congress Control Number: 2018962371

© Springer Nature Switzerland AG 2019
This work is subject to copyright. All rights are reserved by the Publisher, whether the whole or part of the material is concerned, specifically the rights of translation, reprinting, reuse of illustrations, recitation, broadcasting, reproduction on microfilms or in any other physical way, and transmission or information storage and retrieval, electronic adaptation, computer software, or by similar or dissimilar methodology now known or hereafter developed.
The use of general descriptive names, registered names, trademarks, service marks, etc. in this publication does not imply, even in the absence of a specific statement, that such names are exempt from the relevant protective laws and regulations and therefore free for general use.
The publisher, the authors and the editors are safe to assume that the advice and information in this book are believed to be true and accurate at the date of publication. Neither the publisher nor the authors or the editors give a warranty, express or implied, with respect to the material contained herein or for any errors or omissions that may have been made. The publisher remains neutral with regard to jurisdictional claims in published maps and institutional affiliations.

This Springer imprint is published by the registered company Springer Nature Switzerland AG
The registered company address is: Gewerbestrasse 11, 6330 Cham, Switzerland

Foreword

Peritoneal pseudomyxoma and mesothelioma are rare tumors. Despite differences in their pathological structure, these malignancies have some common characteristics, such as lack of reliable diagnostic methods, predominantly peritoneal dissemination, rare lympho-hematogenous metastases, and a difficult choice of optimal treatment strategy. The lack of specific clinical diagnostic symptoms of peritoneal pseudomyxoma and mesothelioma and the rare incidence of these neoplasms cause diagnostic errors; therefore, an accurate interpretation of the histologic results is ultimately needed.

Conventional therapy, such as systemic chemotherapy after diagnostic or symptomatic surgeries of mesothelioma, results in poor prognosis with median of survival of 6–15 months. Systemic therapy of pseudomyxoma peritonei is ineffective, while the volume of completed cytoreduction of pseudomyxoma and mesothelioma is considered to be one of the favorable prognostic factors.

The most effective treatment results may be achieved by the combination of cytoreductive surgery and hyperthermic intraperitoneal chemotherapy (HIPEC). Such approach is universal both for peritoneal pseudomyxoma and mesothelioma. However, a debatable issue is still the search for the most effective regimens of intraperitoneal chemotherapy–hyperthermic chemoperfusion by an "open" or "closed" technique, early postoperative chemotherapy, doses and types of cytostatics, optimal HIPEC temperature, perfusion duration, solution types, as well as the limits of surgical intervention for removing the tumor. The perspective approaches in the treatment of peritoneal pseudomyxoma and mesothelioma are immunotherapies that involve activated and genetically modified lymphocytes and modern target agents including inhibitors of immune checkpoints. All these aspects are covered in detail in the given monograph and will definitely present a helpful tool for clinicians in making differential diagnosis and choosing the treatment strategy for patients with these peritoneal lesions. The material of this book should also encourage research oncologists and molecular biologists in extended studies of carcinogenesis mechanisms of peritoneal pseudomyxoma and mesothelioma in order to search for new diagnostic and prognostic markers, as well as innovative treatment methods of these neoplasms.

Thereby, peritoneal pseudomyxoma and mesothelioma are poorly investigated rare tumors, which require accurate pathological diagnostics, development of a universal examination algorithm, choice of an optimal volume of surgical intervention, and additional methods of treatment. This monograph presents up-to-date conception of etiology, diagnostics, and therapy of peritoneal pseudomyxoma and mesothelioma. The book is designed for a wide audience of students and professors of medical universities and schools, specialists of research and diagnostic centers, practical oncologists and immunologists, as well as doctors of different medical areas.

Moscow, Russia Mikhail I. Davydov

Contents

1 Mesothelioma and Pseudomyxoma peritonei: Incidence, Etiology, Diagnosis 1
Amir G. Abdulaev, Boris E. Polotskiy, and Mikhail M. Davydov

2 Pathology of Selected Primary and Metastatic Tumors of Peritoneum 19
Kozlov A. Nikolay

3 Up to Date Approaches to Treatment of Patients with Pseudomyxoma Peritonei and Peritoneal Mesothelioma 39
Amir G. Abdulaev, Boris E. Polotskiy, and Mikhail M. Davydov

4 Standardizing of Mesothelioma and Pseudomyxoma Care 73
Ranyell Matheus Spencer Sobreira Batista and Thales Paulo Batista

5 Experimental Basis for Optimal Regimnes of Hyperthermic Peritoneal Chemotherapy 91
Natalia Yu. Anisimova, Irina Zh. Zhubina, Fedor V. Donenko, Julia I. Dolzhikova, Antonina V. Kshnaykina, and Mikhail V. Kiselevskiy

6 Immunotherapy of Malignant Peritoneal Mesothelioma and Pseudomyxoma Peritonei 101
Irina Zh. Zhubina, Irina O. Chikileva, and Mikhail V. Kiselevskiy

Index 121

Contributors

Amir G. Abdulaev Oncologist and Surgeon Thoracic Research Department, N.N. Blokhin National Medical Research Center, Moscow, Russia

Natalia Yu. Anisimova Laboratory of Cell Immunity, N.N. Blokhin National Medical Research Center, Moscow, Russia

Ranyell Matheus Spencer Sobreira Batista Department of Pelvic Surgery, AC Camargo Cancer Center, São Paulo, Brazil

Thales Paulo Batista Department of Surgery/Oncology, IMIP, Recife, Recife, Brazil

Department of Surgery, Federal University of Pernambuco, Recife, Brazil

Irina O. Chikileva Laboratory of Cell Immunity, N.N. Blokhin National Medical Research Center, Moscow, Russia

Mikhail M. Davydov Oncologist and Surgeon Thoracic Research Department, N.N. Blokhin National Medical Research Center, Moscow, Russia

Julia I. Dolzhikova Laboratory of Cell Immunity, N.N. Blokhin National Medical Research Center, Moscow, Russia

Fedor V. Donenko Laboratory of Cell Immunity, N.N. Blokhin National Medical Research Center, Moscow, Russia

Mikhail V. Kiselevskiy Laboratory of Cell Immunity, N.N. Blokhin National Medical Research Center, Moscow, Russia

Antonina V. Kshnaykina Laboratory of Cell Immunity, N.N. Blokhin National Medical Research Center, Moscow, Russia

Kozlov A. Nikolay Department of Pathology, N.N. Blokhin National Medical Research Center, Moscow, Russia

Boris E. Polotskiy Oncologist and Surgeon Thoracic Research Department, N.N. Blokhin National Medical Research Center, Moscow, Russia

Irina Zh. Zhubina Laboratory of Cell Immunity, N.N. Blokhin National Medical Research Center, Moscow, Russia

Chapter 1
Mesothelioma and Pseudomyxoma peritonei: Incidence, Etiology, Diagnosis

Amir G. Abdulaev, Boris E. Polotskiy, and Mikhail M. Davydov

Abstract Pseudomyxoma peritonei and peritoneal are similar in predominant affection of peritoneum, low frequency of lymphogenic and hematogenic metastasis and lack of efficient treatment methods. Pseudomyxoma peritonei is a neoplastic disease that is characterized by mucinous carcinomatosis of the peritoneum and it always arises as a result of another tumor of various differentiation grades. Pseudomyxoma peritonei is a rare disease that shows significant difficulties for pathologic differentiation diagnosis from other tumors with intraperitoneal dissemination. Peritoneal mesothelioma (PM) is a primary peritoneal tumor with increasing incidence worldwide. Different histological subtypes with different tumor aggressiveness have been described. Accurate histopathological analysis of an adequate biopsy specimen is needed when a primary peritoneal tumor is suspected. The pattern of spread of PM is predominantly expansive more than infiltrative or haematological.

Keywords Peritoneal mesothelioma · Pseudomyxoma peritonei · Incidence · Etiology · Diagnosis

1.1 Pseudomyxoma peritonei

Pseudomyxoma peritonei (PMP) is a neoplastic disease that is characterized by mucinous carcinomatosis of the peritoneum and it always arises as a result of another tumor of various differentiation grades.

The earliest disease description (a patient with a benign mucocele of the appendix) was presented by Rokitansky in 1842. There is no official statistics of the disease incidence due to an extremely rare occurrence of the tumor; it is generally accepted that annual incidence accounts for 1–2 cases per 1,000,000 people and 1 case of 10,000 laparatomies. Women develop PMP more often than men, Guo et al. report the male/female ratio of 1:3.4 [1].

A. G. Abdulaev (✉) · B. E. Polotskiy · M. M. Davydov
Oncologist and Surgeon Thoracic Research Department, N.N. Blokhin National Medical Research Center, Moscow, Russia

© Springer Nature Switzerland AG 2019

M. V. Kiselevskiy et al. (eds.), *Malignant Mesothelioma and Pseudomyxoma*,
https://doi.org/10.1007/978-3-319-99510-6_1

In some cases intraoperative pseudomyxoma can be recognized as disseminated ovarian cancer, mesothelioma, or colorectal cancer that demonstrates rather complicated clinical diagnostics of the neoplasm. The course of the disease often develops latently with no marked symptoms. The growing tumor masses may cause a moderate pulling pain in the abdomen, body weight loss with decreasing appetite or reduction of the stomach volume due to the external compression. Later the disease inevitably develops to progression and in the end can result in compression of the bowel, ureter, and common bile duct, while clinical condition acquires an acute character.

Literature presents a number of debatable opinions about the origin of pseudomyxoma and its pathologic classification [2–4]. Highly differentiated mucinous tumors of colon, appendiceal adenocarcinoma and mucinous adenocarcinomas originated from any other intraperitoneal organ can have mimic clinical and pathologic characteristics of pseudomyxoma peritonei.

Modern pathologic, molecular-genetic and immunohistochemical data show that in most cases PMP arises from tumors of the appendix [5, 6], which have different biology and prognosis dependent on the differentiation grade. A better prognosis is considered for patients with pseudomyxoma that emerged as a result of the rupture of the mucin producing appendiceal adenoma, rather than mucinous adenocarcinoma [4]. Ronnett et al. showed evidence in favor of this conclusion by their analysis in 1995. The authors studied morphologic characteristics of the removed tumors with pseudomyxoma diagnosis and their prognostic correlation. The researchers divided all cases in three categories: disseminated peritoneal adenomucinosis (DPAM) where the source of pseudomyxoma was low grade malignancies of the appendix; peritoneal mucinous carcinomatosis (PMCA)—if pseudomyxoma progression was associated with low differentiated tumors of the appendix; and, in addition, they separated an intermediate group (IG). An overall 5-year survival was significantly higher in the DPAM category and reached 75%, whereas in PMCA and IG it accounted for 14% and 50%, respectively. Literature analysis shows that the classification proposed by Ronnett et al. makes now the basis for evaluation of survival indexes. The alternative classification was proposed by Carr [7], who also suggested dividing pseudomyxoma cases into groups (G1-G3) on the base of differentiation grades.

On the other hand, some authors consider that a number of PMP cases can have the source of origin such tumors as ovarian, stomach, pancreas, colon, gall bladder, urinary duct, and other intraperitoneal organs [8–11]. Thus, pseudomyxoma peritonei is a rare disease that shows significant difficulties for pathologic differentiation diagnosis from other tumors with intraperitoneal dissemination.

1.1.1 Immuno-pathologic and Molecular-Genetic Diagnosis of Pseudomyxoma peritonei

Pseudomyxoma peritonei is a special condition among secondary peritoneal malignancies. Pseudomyxoma peritonei is a descriptive clinical term and it is used for identification of mucus accumulation on the serosal surface of the abdominal cavity.

Since it is not a diagnosis on its own, it requires differentiation of the primary factor that caused mucus accumulation [7], which often comes from highly differentiated mucinous neoplasms including serrated adenoma, cystadenoma and villous adenoma. Most of these neoplasms are localized in the appendix. The evidence for this fact is established by immunohistochemistry (IHC) that reveals intracellular MUC2 expression—the "intestine" type of mucin in the cells of the mucus secreting epithelium—in these tumors. Fewer cases of pseudomyxoma peritonei refer to the origin from mucinous tumors of colon, pancreas, urachus, gallbladder, and stomach or "mucus forming" tumor of the "appendicular" type, developed within the ovarian teratoma. However, a number of experts consider that in all other cases primary ovarian tumors cannot be the source of pseudomyxoma [7].

Pathologic diagnosis of PMP is rather complicated because of a significant predominance of mucus masses over tumor cells and a large amount of pseudomyxoma surgical material is required to find tumor cells. Yet, it is necessary to determine histologic type of the tumor for disease prognosis. Therefore, to specify the prognosis the pathologic conclusion should include histologic type and the malignancy grade of the tumor, as well as primary organ origin. Tumor elements can present singular cells, small clasters or glandular-like structures floating in the lakes of mucus and containing significant amount of cytoplasmic mucin. Cellular atypia is often minimally expressed, that is characteristic of highly differentiated mucinous neoplasms of low grade malignancy. If "signet ring cell" elements are found, the developing process should be regarded as adenocarcinoma of high grade of malignancy [7].

The researchers also report that IHC analysis of pseudomyxoma tumor cells of appendicular origin not only have "intestine" immunophenotype (CDX2+/CK20+), but also express CK7 in 30% of cases that makes a difference from similar tumors of colorectal localization. Appendicular tumors express CK8, CK18, CK19, MUC2 and DPC4 in the similar way as mucinous adenocarcinomas of colon [12]. Over 80% of appendicular mucinous adenocarcinomas express MUC5AC as their analogue tumors of stomach, pancreas and ovaries do. Furthermore, the cross-expression of CK7+/CK20+ in mucinous tumors in ovaries and appendix implies significant difficulties in differential diagnosis of primary PMP localization [13]. This has led to establishment of the most informative IHC panel including such markers as CK7, CK20, CDX2, MUC2 and MUC5AC. Lack of CK7 expression in parallel with diffuse and intense CK20 expression indicates colorectal localization of primary neoplasm, while CK7+/CK20- phenotype is rather characteristic of primary ovarian cancer [12–14]. In case of simultaneous expression of both markers, evaluation of tumor spreading and stain intensity plays the key role. Diffuse intense CK7 staining with focal expression of CK20 indicates gonadal localization rather than colorectal and *vice versa*. Weak focal expression of transcription factor CDX2, responsible for intestine epithelial differentiation, often occurs in mucinous neoplasms of ovaries and pancreas, which facilitates differential diagnosis from similar tumors of colorectal localization where this marker expression has a clear diffuse character (Fig. 1.1).

Dabbs reports that rare mucinous tumors developing within mature ovarian teratoma have the immunophenotype of lower gastro-intestinal tract parts (CK7-/CK20+/CDX2+) [12]. Differential diagnosis of such neoplasms is based only on

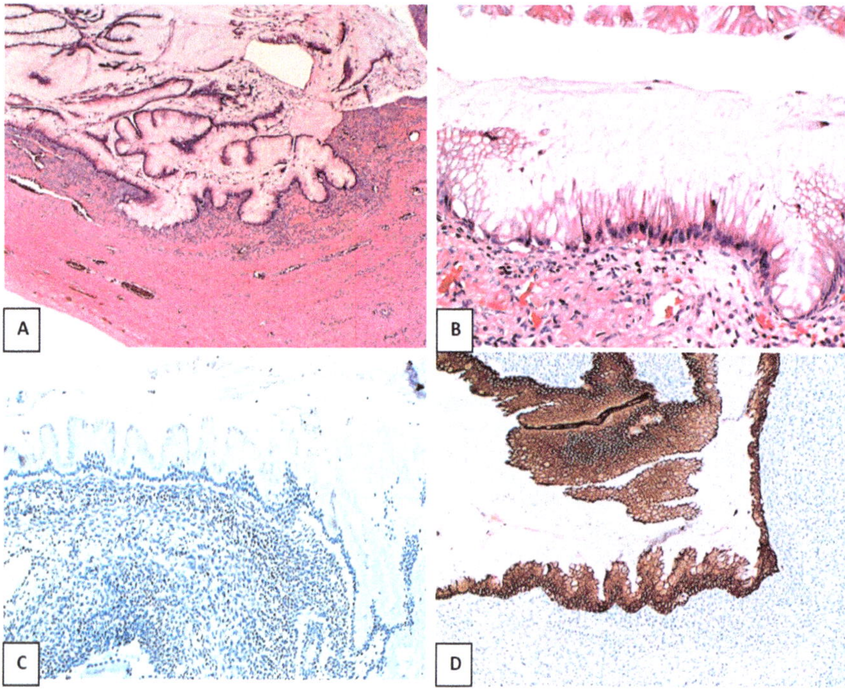

Fig. 1.1 Histological variants of pseudomyxoma peritonei. (**a**) – Pseudomyxoma peritonei, higly differentiated mucinous adenocarcinoma of the appendix, hematoxylin-eosin; (**b**) Pseudomyxoma peritonei, higly differentiated mucinous adenocarcinoma of the appendix, hematoxylin-eosin; (**c**) lack of CK7 expression in tumor cells; (**d**) diffuse cytoplasmatic CK20 expression in tumor cells

clinical pathological data with mandatory exclusion of the primary tumor in gastrointestinal tract. Besides, signet ring cell carcinoma sometimes can cause PMP development and in order to determine the organ of origin it is suggested to use the panel of CK7, CK20, CK5/6, TTF-1, CDX-2, MUC2, ER, PR [14, 15].

Differential diagnosis of PMP also reveals such pathologic processes as endometriosis with myxoidal changes, myxoidal leuomiosarcoma and aggressive angiomyxoma. Despite single cases of mucus forming tumor progression with low differentiation of tumor cells, "classic" type PMP has no invasive potential and does not produce metastases neither hematogenous nor lymphagenous [7]. Another specific feature of pseudomyxoma is its spreading pattern over abdominal cavity. It is generally accepted that it "avoids" serous surface of the intestine, but mainly affects the greater omentum, the right dome of the diaphragm, the right posterior hepatic space, the ligament of Treitz, the right lateral canal, and the pelvic cavity. There are quite a limited number of articles discussing molecular genetic features of pseudomyxoma peritonei. However, they are of great interest and together with immunohisochemical data they help to understand certain specific biological aspects of the tumor, in particular, to reveal the origin of pseudomyxoma peritonei. The conventional method for detection of the tumor origin is immunohistochemistry, however

Table 1.1 Typical profile of expression of mucinous tumors of the intestinal and ovarian origin

IHC marker	Intestinal tumors	Ovarian tumors
CK7	–	+
CK20	+	–
CDX2	+	–
CEA	+	–
MUC1	–	+
MUC2	+	–
MUC5AC	–	+
MUC6	+	–
CA125	–	+
CA19-9	+	–
ER	–	+
PR	–	+

there are no specific IHC markers of pseudomyxoma and IHC profile alone cannot present the unambiguous proof of tumor origin (Table 1.1).

Expression variability of IHC makers may be seen in J.H. Shin and co-authors' report [16], who analyzed immunohistochemical types of 22 mucinous ovarian tumors and 41 metastatic colorectal adenocarcinomas with affected ovaries. The authors describe their markers panel as following: CK7-82.9% of colorectal carcinomas are negative; CK20—65.9% of colorectal carcinomas are diffusively positive, CDX2-73.2% of colorectal adenocarcinomas are positive; CEA—only 41.5% of carcinomas of the intestine origin are positive, MUC2 is expressed in 51.2% of cases, MUC5AC is negative in 97.6% of colorectal tumors, alpha methylacyl-COA racemase (AMACR) is negative in 41.5% of intestinal tumors. However, different authors report different percentage of positive/negative IHC markers expression.

Some authors consider that PMP of the ovarian origin does not exist at all, and pseudomyxoma peritonei may have either unclear involvement of the ovaries in the malignant process or it may be pseudomyxoma with the affected ovaries [1, 11, 17].

Carr et al. (2002) [5] studied pseudomyxoma in 35 females. On the base of the collected data of the IHC panel (CK7, CK20, MUC1, MUC2, CA125, ER, PR) the authors made a conclusion that PMP has appendicular character with possible secondary affected ovaries almost in all cases. Similar conclusion was made by other researchers [17] on the base of a corresponding panel of markers. Szych C. et al. [18] makes the same suggestion, however, taking into account the data on the non-specific—though expressed in a number of tumors—mutations of KRAS gene and deletions in chromosomes 18q, 17p, 5q, and 6q. The problem of primary ovarian tumors of pseudomyxoma peritonei is rather disputable. Besides low specificity of IHC markers, malignant process of progressing tumors of appendicular origin may also involve ovaries. Taflampas P. et al. [19] have analyzed 519 cases of pseudomyxoma of appendicular origin in order to estimate the prognostic role of serum markers CA-125 and CA 19-9 in patients who underwent cytoreduction treatment with hyperthermic intraperitoneal chemotherapy (HIPEC). The researchers show that enhanced serum CA-125, which is commonly associated with ovarian pathologic disorder, as well as "intestinal" CA 19-9 characterizes the course of disease and implies negative connection with disease prognosis [19, 20].

The question is, "Can the protein expression profile change in mucin producing cells after their dissemination over peritoneum and be different from the initial tumor?". Taking into account the fact that the cells enter an unusual microenvironment, such phenomenon may take place. In addition, the data have been reported that demonstrate IHC markers expression alteration determined by the differentiation grade of the mucinous tumors of the appendix [21], which makes it more difficult to establish the tumor histologic origin.

If to consider possible primary origin of pseudomyxoma peritonei from ovarian tumors and secondary involvement of ovaries in the malignant PMP process, it is worth discussing the data presented by Sitzmann J.V. et al. [22]. The authors found the association between hereditary ovarian cancer with BRCA1 and BRCA2 gene mutations and increased incidence of PMP of the appendicular origin. Although BRCA1 and BRCA2 mutations are commonly associated with hereditary breast and ovarian cancers, it should be noted that DNA repair mechanisms, which are aggravated by BRCA, function in the universal manner for all tissues and cells and these mutations increase the risk of emerging tumors of any localization. On the other hand, the difficulty of defining the primary tumor for pseudomyxoma may imply its hereditary syndrome character that is associated with high risk of carcinogenesis of various localizations with predominant colorectal cancer, such as Lynch syndrome and family adenomatosis of the intestine. The logic implies studying mutations and modifications of MLH1, MSH2, MSH6, and PMS2, APC genes and DNA microsatellite instability within this context [23]. However, according to literature data neoplasms of the appendix are just rare cases with hereditary colorectal cancer, while alterations of the given genes and microsatellite instability in appendicular carcinomas have somatic (acquired), but not germ-cell (hereditary) character [23]. No data of hereditary pseudomyxoma have been reported in literature.

Mucinous colorectal tumors being the most probable and frequent origin of pseudomyxoma peritonei present a worse prognosis as compared with non-mucinous tumors [19], which makes it possible to form two groups of markers—markers representing intensity of mucin production by the tumor markers representing differentiation grade and proliferation potential.

One of the most frequent mutations in the gastric-intestinal tumors are KRAS codon 12 gene mutations. Shetty S et al. [24] showed that KRAS codon 12 gene mutations in case of pseudomyxoma were associated with mucin production though have no any impact on overall survival (a cohort of 64 patients). Activating GNAS mutations of highly differentiated appendicular mucinous neoplasms were found in 50% cases (of 36 patients studied) and correlated with mucin production (with MUC2 and MUC5AC expression), but did not affect proliferation rate [25]. F. Mohamed et al. showed in a small cohort that patients' survival has no association with expression of mucins (according to IHC of MUC1 and MUC2) [26]. They analyzed patients with disseminated peritoneal adenomucinosis (pseudomyxoma peritonei of low grade) in two groups—11 cases with malignant disease (median survival of 52.2 months) and 22 cases with no confirmed relapses.

A well-established prognostic factor for pseudomyxoma peritonei is the rate of cell proliferation as well as its differentiation grade [27]. The data representing the fact that molecular makers expression depends not only on histological tumor type, but also on the differentiation grade were reported in a number of studies. Baratti D. et al. [28] made a conclusion that CK20 expression was revealed more often in more differentiated pseudomyxomas (DPAM-disseminated peritoneal adenomucinosis).

Chang MS et al. [21] used immunohistochemistry to study a number of differentiation markers and proteins of cellular activation in 22 mucinous adenomas, 20 mucinous neoplasms with the unknown malignant potential and 14 mucinous adenocarcinomas, and they found that increased expression rates of leptin, MUC2, MUC5AC, mTOR and ERK were associated with tumors of higher malignancy grades. The results showed that disease-free period was significantly shorter in patients with high mTOR expression (11.5 vs 46.7 months, $p = 0.028$). And, as it was mentioned earlier, some data show that high CA-125 and CA 19-9 expression rates are associated with worse survivals in cases of highly differentiated tumors and with a higher risk of relapse, even if a cytoreductive treatment with additional intraperitoneal chemotherapeutic hyperthermia has been performed [19].

Sitzmann JV et al. [22] take into account the data demonstrating that inherited mutations BRCA1 and BRCA2 increase the incidence of pseudomyxoma arising from highly differentiated tumors of appendicular origin and, therefore, the authors suggest considering preventive appendectomy simultaneously with ovarian ectomy if there are any indications.

Another frequent genetic marker is PIK3CK gene mutation that occurs in mucinous tumors of the appendix as well [29]. The researchers have noticed that activating PIK3CK mutations (exones 9 and 20) are found particularly in cecum carcinomas more frequently than in any other parts of the gastro-intestinal tract, which evidently is the specific site for potential disease development [30]. The authors showed that PIK3CK mutations were often associated with KRAS gene mutations (indeed, KRAS mutation is one of the most frequent in colorectal cancers), microsatellite instability and inactivation (methylation) of MGMT gene (DNA repair gene). They also made a conclusion that PIK3CK mutation was associated with a lower overall survival of the patients. Taking into account the literature data and the diverse character of pseudomyxoma peritonei in terms of its biological features and markers, we may suggest that tumor malignancy should be evaluated by integral methods, such as assessment of genome instability rate (microsatellite instability, repair gene and apoptosis inactivation), and measuring activation of intracellular signaling pathways common for many tumors (such as MAPK, PIK3CA, and AKT signaling).

Considering perspectives of target therapy of patients with PMP, Chang MS et al. [21] performed a study of a limited cohort which showed that mucinous tumors had neither Her2 or EGFR amplification, nor ALK rearrangement, although they have high mTOR expression, which makes this molecular marker a potential target for mTOR inhibitor therapy.

Target therapy against PIK3CA, including its combination with mTOR inhibitors [31], may be also quite efficient in pseudomyxoma peritonei taking into consideration a reported predisposition of mucous tumors to PIK3CA gene mutations [29, 30].

Gatalica Z et al. [32] have suggested cycloxygenase-2 (COX2) as additional target for such therapy since these authors have found that COX2 is expressed in tumor cells of pseudomyxoma peritonei and tumor stroma cells of inflammation. The authors believe that COX2 has a good potential in the context of utilizing cyclooxygenase inhibitors.

1.2 Malignant Peritoneal Mesothelioma

In 1908 Miller and Wynn were the first to describe "…a malignant tumor, arising from the peritoneal epithelium and producing mucoid ascitic fluid". On the basis of this description malignant peritoneal mesothelioma (MPM) represents a primary tumor originating from the mesothelial cells of serous membranes (Fig. 1.2). According to the literature data mesothelioma is a rare tumor which incidence is 1–2 cases per one million people with the morbidity of 200–400 patients every year, and incidence rate of pleural mesothelioma is three-fold higher than peritoneal mesothelioma.

Clinical picture of the peritoneal mesothelioma is variable and has no specific features. It often has no symptoms in the early grades; sometimes, a number of patients may have complaints of pains in the abdomen, lack of appetite and weight loss, fever of the unknown reason; possible development of thrombocytosis and hypercoagulability as a result of para-neoplastic syndrome [33]. Later patients' complaints are determined by the localization of the largest lesions, which can lead to a hollow organ compression, mechanical block of the bile ducts or ureter, and intestinal obstruction. Another frequent mesothelioma symptom is malignant ascites. Nevertheless, if a patient refers to a doctor for the first time with complaints about enlarged belly and at examination free liquid is found, an average 4 months will have passed before its exact origin is established [33]. Such fact has several reasons: firstly, mesothelioma of the abdomen is a rare pathologic condition and most doctors have no experience of its diagnosis. Secondly, correct interpretation of the histologic picture and high quality IHC analysis of voluminous material play a

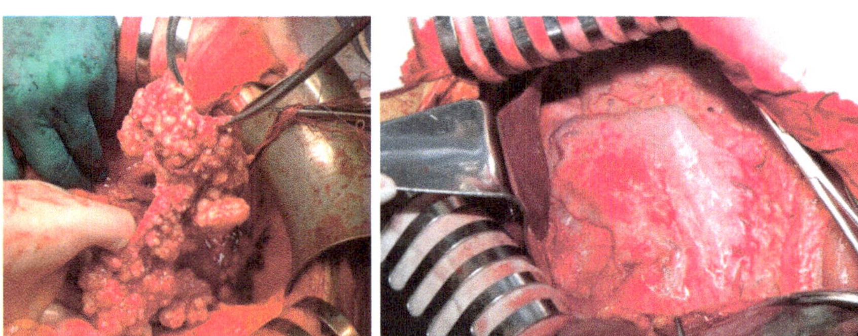

A B

Fig. 1.2 Mesothelioma: (**a**) papillary type; (**b**) epithelioid type very important role, and in connection with that it is necessary, thirdly, to obtain significant tumor amount from biopsy, which is not always easy to do.

According to WHO classification, histologic types of malignant mesothelioma are defined as following:

Epithelioid—75%;
Tubule-papillary solid—13%;
Sarcomatoid—6%;
Biphase—6%.

Besides some reports identify peritoneal mesotheliomas of marginal malignancy that are very rare such as highly differentiated papillary and multicystic variants. Histologic tumor type is considered one of the most significant prognostic factors of peritoneal mesothelioma. And it is noted that patients with highly differentiated papillary and multicystic mesothelioma or epithelioid mesothelioma have a more favorable prognosis than those with sarcomatoid or biphase histologic types.

1.2.1 Etiology and Pathogenesis of Peritoneal Mesothelioma

Etiology of peritoneal mesothelioma is a considerably complicated subject in medicine. As most authors believe the main exogenous factor of this disease is asbestos although the researchers have a lot of discussions concerning mechanisms of its contact with the peritoneum [31, 34, 35]. The researchers report the disease manifestation 20–30 years after the asbestos exposure [36, 37].

A large research [38] was performed in order to study thoroughly any potential mechanisms of influence of the asbestos fibers. The research showed:

Firstly, irritation of the peritoneum by the asbestos fibers can lead to chronic inflammation in the mesothelium which stimulates a permanent process of damaging and reparation that results in release of pro-inflammatory cytokines such as tumor necrosis factor (TNF-α) and reactive oxygen species (ROS). Mesothelial cells exposed to asbestos *in vitro* demonstrated its cytotoxic effect, although it is neutralized by TNF-α which induces nuclear transcription factor NFκB. The latter participates in cell proliferation and apoptosis inhibition [39]. Reactive oxygen species, generated by phagocytic cells such as macrophages and neutrophils, lead to cellular DNA damage and thus potentiate genetic instability and alterations in oncogenes and genes of tumor suppression [40, 41].

Secondly, exposure to asbestos may result in disruption of mitosis due to the destruction of the mitotic fibers, which can be a potential reason for chromosome instability, aneuploidy and other types of chromosomal disorders, which are the base for mesothelioma development [42–44].

Thirdly, anti-apoptotic function of ferritin under asbestos exposure was revealed to inhibit apoptosis in mesothelioma cells. Moreover, ferrous molecules can catalyze ROS formation [45, 46]. Finally, asbestos exposure activates mitogen activated proteinkinase cascades (MAPK), which eventually leads to mesothelioma cell proliferation.

On the other hand, asbestos exposure is not the only etiological factor of developing mesothelioma [47]. In addition, all mineral-based synthetic fibers [48–50], as well as virus SV 40 [51] are considered to be potential inducers of tumor growth in case of prolonged exposure. Carcinogenesis determined by virus SV 40 develops due to the blockade of tumor growth suppressor genes, and Carbone et al. suggested a similar mechanism for development of Non-Hodgkin's [52, 53].

1.2.2 Immuno-pathologic and Molecular-Genetic Diagnostics of Peritoneal Mesothelioma

Histologic analysis of the material obtained with biopsy is performed by a pathologist, and the specialist often has to make a differential diagnosis of mesothelioma, adenocarcinoma and non-epithelial tumors. Therefore, at present immunohistochemical analysis is often used because it enables the most accurate determination of mesothelioma type.

Highly differentiated papillary and diffuse peritoneal mesothelioma types are the most frequently occurring variants of morphologic structure of malignant peritoneal mesothelioma [54]. Typical cases of both types form multiple papillary, simple or complex glandular solid and mixed structures laid with monomorphic population of epithelioid cells with large eosinophilic cytoplasm, clear borders, vesicular nuclei and one or two explicit nucleoli (Fig. 1.3). Specific morphologic feature of highly differentiated papillary mesothelioma is indispensable papillary or tubular-papillary structure that is laid with one layer of cubic or flat cells with minimal atypia and low mitotic activity. In certain cases a marked fibrosis connected with heterogenic location of tumor glandular structures and/or psammomys bodies may lead to a mistake in the diagnosis of malignant mesothelioma and adenocarcinoma [54].

The most important differential diagnostic characteristics of malignant mesothelioma is the presence of invasive foci in the fat tissue of the peritoneal wall or the omentum. However, evaluation of this parameter in the analysis of biopsy material can be rather difficult or even impossible. Potential reason of diagnostic mistake may be the "imbedded" cells of normal mesothelium in the forming granular tissue in chronic inflammatory processes and between fat lobules [54]. Furthermore, reactive mesothelial hyperplasia has no high cellular structure in stromal part of the lesion and it is characterized by zonal arrangement, minimal atypia and extremely rare necrotic areas [55].

Diffuse mesothelioma type may be mistakenly diagnosed because of its macro- and microscopic growth specificity and wrongly considered either as secondary lesion or primary serous peritoneal cancer. After histochemical staining malignant mesothelioma cells reveal acid mucins (hyaluronic acid), while adenocarcinoma typically reveals neutral mucins. The reports show that typical malignant mesothelioma cells present synchronous expression of vimentin, thrombomodulin, calretinin, caldesmon, D2-40 and cytokeratins with the lack of expression of other

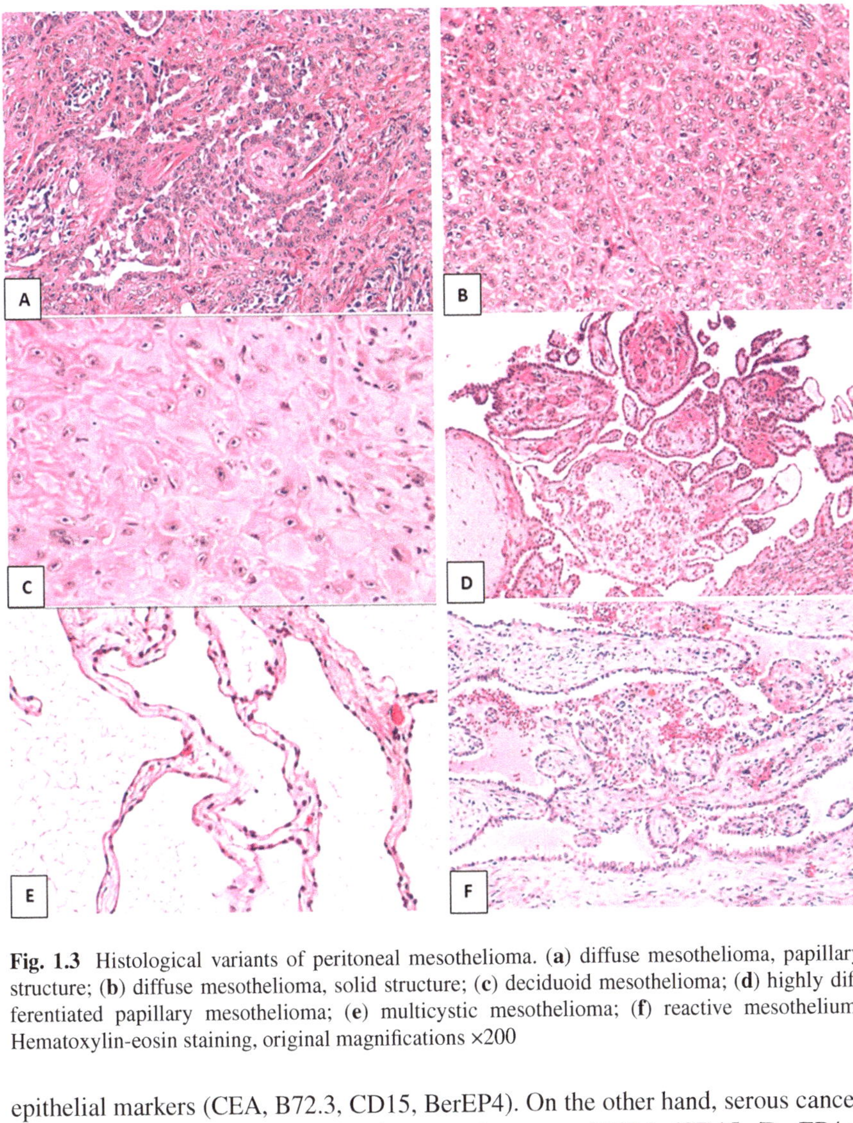

Fig. 1.3 Histological variants of peritoneal mesothelioma. (**a**) diffuse mesothelioma, papillary structure; (**b**) diffuse mesothelioma, solid structure; (**c**) deciduoid mesothelioma; (**d**) highly differentiated papillary mesothelioma; (**e**) multicystic mesothelioma; (**f**) reactive mesothelium. Hematoxylin-eosin staining, original magnifications ×200

epithelial markers (CEA, B72.3, CD15, BerEP4). On the other hand, serous cancer is characterized by the opposite immunophenotype (B72.3+/CD15+/BerEP4+/CA19-9+/ER+/calretinin-/caldesmon-/thrombomodulin-) regardless of organ location [14]. It is important to note, that at present there is no any specific mesothelioma marker. Clement emphasizes that due to such fact mesothelioma diagnostics requires consideration not only immunohistochemical results but also the data from light microscopy and histochemistry [56]. The most sensitive markers of all mesothelioma diagnostic range are considered calretinin and BerEP4 [54]. Summarized data of the immunophenotypic features of differential diagnostics of malignant mesothelioma are shown in Table 1.2 [14, 55, 57].

Table 1.2 Immunohistochemic markers for differential diagnostics of malignant mesothelioma

Marker	Mesothelioma	Adenocarcinoma
Vimetin	+	±
Pan-cytokeratin	+	+
Cytokeratin 5/6	+	−
Epithelial membrane antigen, membrane cytoplasm cancer embryonic antigen	−	+
CD15 (Leu-M1)	−	+
Ber-EP4	± (25%)	+
E-cadherin	−	+
B72.3	−	+
MOC-31	−	+
Calretinin	+	−
Thrombomodulin	+	−
Mesothelin	+	−
HMBE-1	+	−
WT-1	+	±
D2–40	+	−

Highly differentiated papillary mesothelioma is reported to have no cellular stratification, complex papillary architecture and mixed cell population, which are typical for serous tumors of low malignancy grade; it is also devoid of high mitotic function and marked atypia that is characteristic of serous cancer. The latter feature helps differentiate highly differentiated papillary mesothelioma from diffuse malignant mesothelioma, that has a more marked atypia. The absence of previous abdominal surgeries or inflammatory processes in the anamnesis and detected papillary structures allow differentiation of highly differentiated papillary mesothelioma from reactive hyperplasia of mesothelium [54].

Another type of slowly progressing mesothelial tumor that needs differential diagnostics is multicystic mesothelioma (synonym, multimodal inclusive peritoneal cyst). The latter develops more often in young or middle-aged women, is not associated with asbestos, has a variable biological potential, spreads over peritoneum without invasive growth and forms multiple thin wall cysts filled with translucent liquid.

Clement et al. [58] suggests that in certain cases cystic lymphangioma can imitate multicystic peritoneal mesothelioma. Nevertheless, the first one is more frequent in children and male adolescents, more often has an external pelvic localization, lying in the mesentery slim and colon, the great omentum, or retroperitoneum [56] (Fig. 1.3).

Secondary or reactive mesothelial hyperplasia in some cases may be a reason of diagnostic error in the analysis of biopsy material of small amount. Reactive hyperplasia of mesothelium is a stereotypic reaction to chronic inflammation or peritoneal ascites and it is frequently found by microscopic analysis as single or multiple proliferative areas on the peritoneum in the site of the appendages in chronic salpingitis, or endometriosis, in large omentum - in case of ovarian tumors,—in the hernia wall or in the site of laparoscopic intervention [55, 56].

Most of literature data about molecular characteristics of mesothelioma refer to pleural mesothelioma since its higher incidence rate. Nevertheless, literature analysis demonstrates that peritoneal mesothelioma has molecular specific features and cannot be always compared with pleural mesothelioma in terms of molecular genetic description. In particular, the analysis of the data of mesotheliomas of different origin in the catalogue of mutations COSMIC shows significant differences in mutation profiles.

Despite a small number of samples of peritoneal mesothelioma listed in the database, one can see that the main genetically significant difference between pleural mesothelioma and peritoneal mesothelioma is the frequency of mutations of EGFR gene encoding epidermal growth factor receptor. The frequency of the revealed mutations activating EGFR kinase domain in pleural mesothelipma accounts for only 2% [57], while Foster et al., found activating EGFR mutations in 9 (31%) out of 29 samples of peritoneal mesothelioma [58].

Activating EGFR gene mutations have no reliable connection with the expression of EGFR protein and amplification of the chromosome site with EGFR gene. Enomoto et al. analyzed by IHC 22 cases of pleural mesothelioma and 16 peritoneal mesotheliomas and found neither correlation between mesothelioma peculiar origin and EGFR expression nor connection between EGFR gene amplification (FISH analysis) and EGFR protein expression [59].

The issue of EGFR mutation status in mesothelioma is still disputable and rather controversial [60], maybe due to difficulties in performing wide-range trials because of rare occurrence of the tumor.

Since Foster et al. Showed high frequency (31%) of activating EGFR mutations in patients with peritoneal mesothelioma [58], it is possible to consider treatment with EGFR target agents. The same authors carried out an *in vitro* research on the cell culture with transfection of the mutant EGFR and showed a potential effectiveness of Erlotinib for treatment of patients with peritoneal mesothelioma and EGFR activating mutations. It is essential that the types and frequency of the revealed mutations are significantly different from the range of EGFR gene mutations of lung adenocarcinoma where molecular genetic analysis for EGFR mutations has already become a standard laboratory procedure in clinics.

Despite these promising data, a team of other researchers [60] made an opposite conclusion—no EGFR activating mutations were found in cell cultures of 33 peritoneal mesotheliomas and therefore, the authors called into question feasibility of anti-EGFR therapy.

Perhaps, target approach to the treatment of mesotheliomas could be similar to that which is used in other tumors of epithelial origin due to frequent cellular activation of signaling pathways MAPK и PI3K/AKT [61, 62] typical to epithelial tumors, including autocrine mechanism [53].

Regarding genetic specificity of different mesothelioma types, it is necessary to note that authors reported just single cases of hereditary mesotheliomas associated with germ cell mutations of the gene BAP1 (BRCA-associated protein 1) [63]. Mutations are revealed in 10% of sporadic mesotheliomas [64], though, certainly, the frequency of germ cell mutations depends on the population.

1.2.3 Differential Diagnosis of Peritoneal Mesothelioma by Molecular Methods

Qualitative and quantitative differences in the expression of different types of proteins make a characteristic profile of each type of cells and tissues. At present immunohistochemistry (IHC) is a routine method which enables to reveal a number of important diagnostic details. The studies have not found any pathognomonic IHC marker for mesothelioma [65, 66]. It is established that at least two positive and two negative markers are required to confirm the diagnosis, and the antibody panel is determined by the exact differential diagnostic purpose. The examples of selectively used antibodies are given in Table 1.3. The specific feature of peritoneal mesothelioma unlike pleural mesothelioma is a crucial importance of differential diagnostics from metastatic tumors originating from peritoneal organs. (Table 1.3).

Moreover, IHC methods are considered difficult to standardize and a significant variability is reported among different laboratories that is caused by different antibody clones, and especially be specific techniques of material processing, which makes every laboratory validate IHC panels according to its conditions. The recommended mesothelioma markers sensitivity should be not less than 80% taking into account the antibodies used in the panel [65].

A number of factors determine disease prognosis of mesothelioma and the most significant of them (as in many other malignancies) are proliferation and invasion character, and metastatic potential. These characteristics are determined mainly by the mesothelioma histologic type.

IHC evaluates prognostic molecular markers such as proliferation marker Ki67 and anti-apoptotic protein BCL-2. K. Pillai et al. Performed a study involving 42 patients with peritoneal mesothelioma and as a result they made a conclusion that

Table 1.3 Differential diagnostic IHC panels

Differential diagnostic case	Panel of antibodies	References
Benign mesothelial proliferation/mesothelioma	Desmin (+)/p53 (+); EMA (+)	[38, 39]
Metastatic carcinomas of gastrointestinal tract/mesothelioma	CEA, MOC-31, CDX-2	[22, 32]
Serous ovarian cancer/mesothelioma	ER, Ber-EP4, PAX8, PAX2, B72.3	[23, 25]
Metastatic renal carcinoma/mesothelioma	Claudine 4, PAX2, PAX8	[35, 36]
Lymphoma, large-cell carcinoma/mesothelioma	CD45 (LCA), CD20 or CD30	[38]
Melanoma/mesothelioma	S100; HMB-45	[38]
Angiosarcoma, epithelioid hemangioendothelioma/mesothelioma	CD31; CD34 Together with positive markers of mesothelioma-calretinin, D2-40, CK5/6, WT1, EMA, mesothelin, thrombomodulin h-CD (h-caldesmon), HBME-1.	[38]

Ki67-BCL2 index was a significant prognostic parameter [67]. Another research showed that BCL2 high expression was a favorable prognostic factor [68].

1.3 Conclusion

Therefore, IHC and molecular genetic data show that peritoneal mesothelioma has a number of differences with pleural mesothelioma including molecular specific features, which makes it separate type of mesothelioma. The task of crucial importance is differential diagnostics of peritoneal mesothelioma from secondary peritoneal lesions. Due to rare cases peritoneal mesothelioma molecular profile is not well described, although EGFR hyperexpression is one of the key mechanisms of tumor pathogenesis. In general, the literature description of molecular changes are not specific and they are characteristic for many epithelial tumors, however, they may be set as the basic point for planning target therapy, in particular, by anti-EGFR drugs. Different histological subtypes with different tumour aggressiveness have been described. Accurate histopathological analysis of an adequate biopsy specimen is needed when a primary peritoneal tumour is suspected. The pattern of spread of PM is predominantly expansive more than infiltrative or haematological. So, it is important to note, that tumor-related individual immunocytochemic molecular-genetic characteristics may have an essential impact on the course of the disease. The analysis of rare mucinous tumors that initiate development of pseudomyxoma peritonei may be especially valuable with this regard. At present, a range of morphological and genetic parameters is being collected into a wide panel that will characterize a tumor in terms of its origin, differentiation grade, and its potential for target therapy.

References

1. Guo AT, Song X, Wei LX, Zhao P (2011) Histological origin of pseudomyxoma peritonei in Chinese women: clinicopathology and immunohistochemistry. World J Gastroenterol 17(30):3531–3537
2. Misdraji J, Yantiss RK, Graeme-Cook FM, Balis UJ, Young RH (2003) Appendiceal mucinous neoplasms: a clinicopathologic analysis of 107 cases. Am J Surg Pathol 27:1089–1103
3. Moran BJ, Cecil TD (2003) The etiology, clinical presentation, and management of pseudomyxoma peritonei. Surg Oncol Clin N Am 12:585–603
4. Nakakura EK (2012) Pseudomyxoma peritonei: more questions than answers. J Clin Oncol 30(20):2429–2430
5. Carr NJ, Emory TS, Sobin LH (2002) Epithelial neoplasms of the appendix and colorectum: an analysis of cell proliferation, apoptosis and expression of p53, CD44, bcl-2. Arch Pathol Lab Med 126:837–841
6. Ronnett BM, Zahn CM, Kurman RJ, Kass ME, Sugarbaker PH, Shmookler BM (1995) Disseminated peritoneal adenomucinosis and peritoneal mucinous carcinoma¬tosis: a clinicopathologic analysis of 109 cases with emphasis on distinguishing pathologic features, site of origin, prognosis and relationship to pseudomyxoma peritonei. Am J Surg Pathol 19:1390–1408

7. Carr NJ, Emory TS, Sobin LH (2003) Epithelial neoplasms of the appendix. In: Odze RD, Goldblum RG (eds) Surgical pathology of the GI tract, liver, biliary tract and pancreas. IARC Press, Lyon, pp 645–647
8. Imaoka H, Yamao K, Salem AA, Mizuno N, Takahashi K, Sawaki A, Isaka T, Okamoto Y, Yanagisawa A, Shimizu Y (2006) Pseudomyxoma peritonei caused by acute pancreatitis in intraductal papillary mucinous carcinoma of the pancreas. Pancreas 32(2):223–224
9. Hawes D, Robinson R, Wira R (1991) Pseudomyxoma peritonei from metastatic colloid carcinoma of the breast. Gastrointest Radiol 16:80–82
10. Kahn MA, Demopoulos RI (1992) Mucinous ovarian tumors with pseudomyxoma peritonei: a clinicopathological study. Int J Gynecol Pathol 11:15–23
11. Ronnett BM, Seidman JD (2003) Mucinous tumors arising in ovarian mature cystic teratomas: relationship to the clinical syndrome of pseudomyxoma peritonei. Am J Surg Pathol 27:650–657
12. Dabbs DJ (ed) (2010) Diagnostic immunohistochemistry: theranostic and genomic applications. Saunders, Philadelphia, pp 511–648
13. Vang R, Ronnett BM (2009) Metastatic and miscellaneous tumors of the ovary. In: Nucci MR, Oliva E (eds) Gynecologic pathology. Elsevier, Edinburgh, pp 539–564
14. Bahrami A, Luan DT, Jae YR (2008) Undifferentiated tumor: true identity by immunohistochemistry. Arch Pathol Lab Med 132:326–348
15. Terada T (2013) An immunohistochemical study of primary signet-ring cell carcinoma of the stomach and colorectum: expression of EMA, CEA, CA19-9, CDX-2, p53, Ki-67 antigen, TTF-1 and p63 in normal mucosa and in 42 cases. Int J Clin Exp Pathol 6(4):630–638
16. Shin JH, Bae JH, Lee A, Jung CK, Yim HW, Park JS, Lee KY (2010) CK7, CK20, CDX2 and MUC2 Immunohistochemical staining used to distinguish metastatic colorectal carcinoma involving ovary from primary ovarian mucinous adenocarcinoma. Jpn J Clin Oncol 40(3):208–213
17. Ferreira CR, Carvalho JP, Soares FA, Siqueira SA, Carvalho FM (2008) Mucinous ovarian tumors associated with pseudomyxoma peritonei of adenomucinosis type: immunohistochemical evidence that they are secondary tumors. Int J Gynecol Cancer 18(1):59–65
18. Szych C, Staebler A, Connolly DC, Wu R, Cho KR, Ronnett BM (1999) Molecular genetic evidence supporting the clonality and appendiceal origin of Pseudomyxoma peritonei in women. Am J Pathol 154(6):1849–1855
19. Taflampas P, Dayal S, Chandrakumaran K, Mohamed F, Cecil TD, Moran BJ (2014) Preoperative tumour marker status predicts recurrence and survival after complete cytoreduction and hyperthermic intraperitoneal chemotherapy for appendiceal Pseudomyxoma Peritonei: analysis of 519 patients. Eur J Surg Oncol 40(5):515–520
20. Baratti D, Kusamura S, Nonaka D, Cabras AD, Laterza B, Deraco M (2009) Pseudomyxoma peritonei: biological features are the dominant prognostic determinants after complete cytoreduction and hyperthermic intraperitoneal chemotherapy. Ann Surg 249(2):243–249
21. Chang MS, Byeon SJ, Yoon SO, Kim BH, Lee HS, Kang GH, Kim WH, Park KJ (2012) Leptin, MUC2 and mTOR in appendiceal mucinous neoplasms. Pathobiology 79(1):45–53
22. Sitzmann JV, Wiebke EA (2013) Risk-reducing appendectomy and the elimination of BRCA1-associated intraperitoneal cancer. JAMA Surg 148(3):285–291
23. Taggart MW, Galbincea J, Mansfield PF, Fournier KF, Royal RE, Overman MJ, Rashid A, Abraham SC (2013) High-level microsatellite instability in appendiceal carcinomas. Am J Surg Pathol 37(8):1192–1200
24. Shetty S, Thomas P, Ramanan B, Sharma P, Govindarajan V, Loggie B (2013) Kras mutations and p53 overexpression in pseudomyxoma peritonei: association withphenotype and prognosis. J Surg Res 180(1):97–103
25. Nishikawa G, Sekine S, Ogawa R, Matsubara A, Mori T, Taniguchi H, Kushima R, Hiraoka N, Tsuta K, Tsuda H, Kanai Y (2013) Frequent GNAS mutations in low-grade appendiceal mucinous neoplasms. Br J Cancer 108(4):951–958

26. Mohamed F, Gething S, Haiba M, Brun EA, Sugarbaker PH (2004) Clinically aggressive pseudomyxoma peritonei: a variant of a histologically indolent process. J Surg Oncol 86(1):10–15
27. van Ruth S, Acherman YI, van de Vijver MJ, Hart AA, Verwaal VJ, Zoetmulder FA (2003) Pseudomyxoma peritonei: a review of 62 cases. Eur J Surg Oncol 29(8):682–688
28. Baratti D, Kusamura S, Nonaka D, Langer M, Andreola S, Favaro M, Gavazzi C, Laterza B, Deraco M (2008) Pseudomyxoma peritonei: clinical pathological and biological prognostic factors in patients treated with cytoreductive surgery and hyperthermic intraperitoneal chemotherapy (HIPEC). Ann Surg Oncol 15(2):526–534
29. Pulighe F, Paliogiannis P, Cossu A, Palmieri G, Colombino M, Scognamillo F, Trignano M (2013) Molecular analysis of appendiceal mucinous cystadenoma and rectal adenocarcinoma in a patient with urothelial carcinoma: a case report. J Med Case Rep 7(1):170
30. Zou Y, Wang F, Liu FY, Huang MZ, Li W, Yuan XQ, Huang OP, He M (2013) RNF43 RNF43 mutations are recurrent in Chinese patients with mucinous ovarian carcinoma but absent in other subtypes of ovarian cancer. Gene 531(1):112–116
31. Green FL, Page DL, Fleming ID et al (2002) AJCC cancer staging handbook. From: AJCC cancer staging manual, 6th edn. Springer, New York, pp 205–209
32. Gatalica Z, Loggie B (2006) COX-2 expression in pseudomyxoma peritonei. Cancer Lett 244(1):86–90
33. De Pangher Manzini V (2005) Malignant peritoneal mesothelioma. Tumori 91:1–5
34. Friedberg JS (2001) Chapter 56 pleura: anatomy, physiology and disorders. In: Norton JF, Bollinger RR, Chang AE et al (eds) Surgery: basic science and clinical evidence. Springer, New York, pp 1243–1264
35. Boylon AM, Broaddus CV (2005) Tumors of the peura. In: Mason RJ, Broaddus VC, Murray JF et al (eds) Textbook of respiratory medicine, 4th edn. Elsevier Saunders, Philadelphia
36. Nepomnyashchaya EM, Bosenko SP (2001) Malignant pleural mesothelioma. Pulmonology 1:65–68
37. Aisner J, Wiernik PN (1978) Malignant mesothelioma: current status and future prospects. Chest 74:438–444
38. Welch LS, Acherman YIZ, Haile E et al (2005) Asbestos and peritoneal mesothelioma among college-educated men. Int J Occup Environ Health 11:254–258
39. Yang H, Bocchetta M, Kroczynska B et al (2006) TNF-alpha inhibits asbestos-induced cytotoxicity via a NF-kappaB-dependent pathway, a possible mechanism for asbestos-induced oncogenesis. Proc Natl Acad Sci 103:10397–10402
40. Shatos MA, Doherty JM, Marsh JP et al (1987) Prevention of asbestosinduced cell death in rat lung fibroblasts and alveolar macrophages by scavengers of active oxygen species. Environ Res 44:103–116
41. Moyer VD, Cistulli CA, Vaslet CA et al (1994) Oxygen radicals and asbestos carcinogenesis. Environ Health Perspect 102(Suppl 10):131–136
42. Ault JG, Cole RW, Jensen CG et al (1995) Behavior of crocidolite asbestos during mitosis in living vertebrate lung epithelial cells. Cancer Res 55:792–798
43. Topov J, Kolev K (1987) Cytology of experimental mesotheliomas induced with crocidolite asbestos. Acta Cytol 31:369–373
44. Craighead JE, Akley NJ, Gould LB et al (1987) Characteristics of tumors and tumor cells cultured from experimental asbestos-induced mesotheliomas in rats. Am J Pathol 129:448–462
45. Aung W, Hasegawa S, Furukawa T et al (2007) Potential role of ferritin heavy chain in oxidative stress and apoptosis in human mesothelial and mesothelioma cells: implications for asbestos-induced oncogenesis. Carcinogenesis 28:2047–2052
46. Kamp DW, Israbian VA, Preusen SE et al (1995) Asbestos causes DNA strand breaks in cultured pulmonary epithelial cells: role of ironcatalyzed free radicals. Am J Phys 268:471–480
47. Kashansky SV, Shaburov AP (2005) Pleural mesothelioma and asbestos exposure. Mater. XVII Sverdlovsk region. Conference on oncologists. Ekaterinburg, pp. 273–276; Kogan FM (1997) White book on white asbestos (chrysotile). Ekaterinburg 71

48. Vasilyeva LA, Pylev LN, Pivovarova LN et al (1991) Carcinogenic and fibrogenic activity of synthetic amphibole asbestos with different chemical structure. Exp Oncol 13:12–15
49. Baris YI (1981) Malignant mesothelioma and radiological chest abnormalities in two villages in Central Turkey. An epidemiological and environmental investigations. Lancet 1:984–987
50. Belitsky GA (2006) Chemical carcinogenesis. Probl Clin Med 1(5):10–15
51. Vilchez RA, Kozinetz CA, Arrington AS et al (2003) Simian virus 40 in human cancers. Am J Med 114:675–684
52. Carbone M, Fisher S, Powers A et al (1999) New molecular and epidemiological issues in mesothelioma: role of SV 40. J Cell Physiol 180:167–172
53. Carbone M, Pass HI, Rizzo P et al (1994) Simian virus 40 large—tantigen binds p 53 in human mesotheliomas. Nat Med 3:908–912
54. Mok SC, Schorge JO, Weich WR et al (2003) Peritoneal tumours. In: Tavassoli FA, Devilee P (eds) World Health Organization classification of tumours. Pathology & genetics of tumours of breast and female genital organs. IARC Press, Lyon, pp 197–202
55. Weiss SW, Goldblum JR (eds) (2008) Enzinger and Weiss's soft tissue tumors, 5th edn. Mosby Elsevier, Philadelphia, pp 789–817
56. Clement PB, Young RH (2010) The peritoneum. In: Mills SE (ed) Sternberg's diagnostic surgical pathology, 5th edn. Lippincott Williams & Wilkins, pp 2393–2412
57. Jänne PA, Wozniak AJ, Belani CP, Keohan ML, Ross HJ, Polikoff JA et al (2005) Open-label study of pemetrexed alone or in combination with cisplatin for the treatment of patients with peritoneal mesothelioma: outcomes of an expanded access program. Clin Lung Cancer 7(1):40–46
58. Foster JM, Radhakrishna U, Govindarajan V, Carreau JH, Gatalica Z, Sharma P et al (2010) Clinical implications of novel activating EGFR mutations in malignant peritoneal mesothelioma. World J Surg Oncol 8:88
59. Enomoto Y, Kasai T, Takeda M, Takano M, Morita K, Kadota E et al (2012) A comparison of epidermal growth factor receptor expression in malignant peritoneal and pleural mesothelioma. Pathol Int 62(4):226–231
60. Kalra N, Ashai A, Xi L, Zhang J, Avital I, Raffeld M et al (2012) Patients with peritoneal mesothelioma lack epidermal growth factor receptor tyrosine kinase mutations that would make them sensitive to tyrosine kinase inhibitors. Oncol Rep 27(6):1794–1800
61. López-Lago MA, Okada T, Murillo MM, Socci N, Giancotti FG (2009) Loss of the tumor suppressor gene NF2, encoding merlin, constitutively activates integrin-dependent mTORC1 signaling. Mol Cell Biol 29(15):4235–4249
62. Turner K, Varghese S, Alexander HR Jr (2012) Current concepts in the evaluation and treatment of patients with diffuse malignant peritoneal mesothelioma. J Natl Compr Cancer Netw 10(1):49–57
63. Ribeiro C, Campelos S, Moura CS, Machado JC, Justino A, Parente B (2013) Well-differentiated papillary mesothelioma: clustering in a Portuguese family with a germline BAP1 mutation. Ann Oncol 24(8):2147–2150
64. Testa JR, Cheung M, Pei J, Below JE, Tan Y, Sementino E, Cox NJ, Dogan AU, Pass HI, Trusa S, Hesdorffer M, Nasu M, Powers A, Rivera Z, Comertpay S, Tanji M, Gaudino G, Yang H, Carbone M (2011) Germline BAP1 mutations predispose to malignant mesothelioma. Nat Genet 43(10):1022–1025
65. Husain AN, Colby TV, Ordóñez NG, Krausz T, Borczuk A, Cagle PT et al (2009) Guidelines for pathologic diagnosis of malignant mesothelioma: a consensus statement from the International Mesothelioma Interest Group. Arch Pathol Lab Med 133(8):1317–1331
66. Marchevsky AM (2008) Application of immunohistochemistry to the diagnosis of malignant mesothelioma. Arch Pathol Lab Med 132(3):397–401
67. Pillai K, Pourgholami MH, Chua TC, Morris DL (2013) Ki67-BCL2 index in prognosis of malignant peritoneal mesothelioma. Am J Cancer Res 3(4):411–423
68. Pillai K, Pourgholami MH, Chua TC, Morris DL (2013) Does the expression of BCL2 have prognostic significance in malignant peritoneal mesothelioma? Am J Cancer Res 3(3):312–322

Chapter 2
Pathology of Selected Primary and Metastatic Tumors of Peritoneum

Kozlov A. Nikolay

Abstract Tumor pathology of the peritoneum is a vast field of activity for a practicing surgical pathologist. The variety of neoplastic lesions of the serous lining of the abdominal cavity is one of the most extensive in the diagnostic pathology. The tasks that the clinician poses for pathologist include not only verifying the pathological diagnosis of the tumor, but also determining the grade of malignancy, organ of origin, distinguishing of malignant and reactive processes. Successful solution of these tasks by a pathologist is a corner-stone of patient management, effectiveness of therapy, and finally, the survival of the patient. This chapter covers a number of rare pathological processes of the peritoneum, which sometimes can create significant diagnostic difficulties for pathologists.

Keywords Malignant mesothelioma · Pseudomyxoma peritonei · Mesothelial lesions · Peritoneal carcinomatosis · Prognosis

2.1 Primary Mesothelial Lesions of the Peritoneum

Practical pathologists often encounter primary and metastatic tumors and tumor-like lesions of abdominal cavity in addition to a wide spectrum of inflammatory lesions of the peritoneum. Therefore, it is of great importance for surgical pathologists to be familiar both with specific tumor types arising from serosal lining of abdominal cavity and with secondary tumors and tumor-like peritoneal lesions. Pathological classification of peritoneal mesothelial neoplasms is presented in Table 2.1.

K. A. Nikolay (✉)
Department of Pathology, N.N. Blokhin National Medical Research Center, Moscow, Russia

© Springer Nature Switzerland AG 2019

M. V. Kiselevskiy et al. (eds.), *Malignant Mesothelioma and Pseudomyxoma*, https://doi.org/10.1007/978-3-319-99510-6_2

Table 2.1 Histopathological classification of primary mesothelial tumors of the peritoneum [WHO 2014]

Histological entity	Code	Biological potential
Adenomatoid tumor	9054/0	Benign tumor
Well-differentiated papillary mesothelioma	9052/0	Benign tumor
Malignant mesothelioma	9050/3	Malignant tumor
epithelioid		
biphasic		
sarcomatoid		

2.1.1 Pathobiology of Mesothelial Tumor and Tumor-Like Lesions of the Peritoneum

Despite the fact that the adenomatoid tumor (AT), well-differentiated papillary mesothelioma (WDPM) and malignant mesothelioma (MM) are not distinguishable from pleural analogues in their morphological, histochemical and immunohistochemical features, mesothelial tumors of the peritoneum have a number of specific clinico-pathological and molecular features. Thus, peritoneal MM has a much lower incidence of biphasic and sarcomatoid variants of the tumor compared with pleural MM [1, 2]. Unlike their pleural analogues, the frequency of peritoneal AT and WDPM is much higher. In most cases, peritoneal MM, in contrast to its pleural analogue, does not demonstrate homozygous p16 deletion, but has a stable loss of immunohistochemical expression of BAP1.

2.1.1.1 Adenomatoid Tumor

Definition Rare benign tumor of mesothelial origin.

Epidemiology and Clinical Features AT can develop at any age, but most often it is observed in middle-aged and elderly women. As a rule, AT is detected accidentally during surgical procedures for other pathological lesions. The most common site of involvement is a serous lining of the fallopian tubes (AT is one of the most common benign tubal tumors) [3], ovaries, and intramural foci in myometrium. Fewer lesions develop in the omentum or gut mesentery [4].

Gross Pathology Macroscopic examination demonstrates small dense nodules with a circumferential border situated directly under the tubal serous membrane or located intramuraly in myometrium. The tumor without a capsule but with a clear border not exceeding 2 cm in diameter is defined on the section. Unlike most leiomyomas AT cannot be extracted from the surrounding tissues (invasive growth) [3, 5]. Cystic transformation of individual larger nodules may develop in rare cases [4].

Histopathology The tumor is represented by infiltrative growth of anastomosing cells with signs of mesothelial differentiation, cytoplasmic vacuoles and cytologically benign round to oval nuclei without nucleoli, and extremely rare mitotic figures. Neoplastic cells are organized in typical for AT lace-like anastomizing tubular and angiomatoid structures. The latter can be represented by both slit-like spaces and signet ring-like cells with large empty vacuoles in the cytoplasm, which often makes a misleading impression of the vascular histogenesis of the neoplasm [3, 5] (Fig. 2.1).

The shape of the described structures can vary in one lesion from rounded-oval to slit-shaped with pointed edges; some of these can be cystically dilated. Homogeneous basophilic content is often observed in the lumen of glandular-like spaces. The lining of the described above structures is represented by cytologically benign cells of a cuboidal or flattened form, with minimal or undetectable mitotic activity. The second most frequent growth pattern is a solid variant of tumor, presented by layers of tumor cells with abundant eosinophilic cytoplasm [4]. In some cases, there are well-defined papillary structures in the tumor. The above-described gland-like and vascular-like spaces are lined by cuboidal or flattened cells. Despite the benign course of disease, microscopic examination shows the infiltrative nature of growth with spreading of cells among smooth muscle fibers.

Immunophenotype Adenomatoid tumor is diffusely positive for PanCK, CK5/6, vimentin, WT-1, calretinin, HBME-1 and thrombomodulin [4], and demonstrate negative expression of vascular markers [6].

Differential Diagnosis AT should be differentiated from primary or metastatic carcinomatous lesions of the peritoneum and vascular neoplasms [4]. Although AT, unlike cancer, has no cellular and nuclear atypia and has minimal mitotic activity, differential diagnosis requires immunohistochemical study in difficult cases, confirming mesothelial differentiation of the tumor cells and the absence of cytological signs of MM [7]. Unlike histologically similar lipoleiomyoma, AT demonstrates a distinguishing expression of mesothelial markers.

Prognosis AT has favorable prognosis.

2.1.1.2 Well-Differentiated Papillary Mesothelioma

Definition well-differentiated tumor of mesothelial origin with papillary growth pattern and indolent clinical behavior.

Epidemiology WDPM affects more often the peritoneum than the pleura, develops more often in women, where it affects mostly the pelvic peritoneum. Development of WDPM is not associated with the asbestos.

Clinical Course The tumor is often detected accidentally. WDPM is characterized by a protracted non-aggressive course of disease.

Gross Pathology WDPM typically manifests as multiple small nodules on the surface of the peritoneum, usually not exceeding 2 cm in the largest dimension.

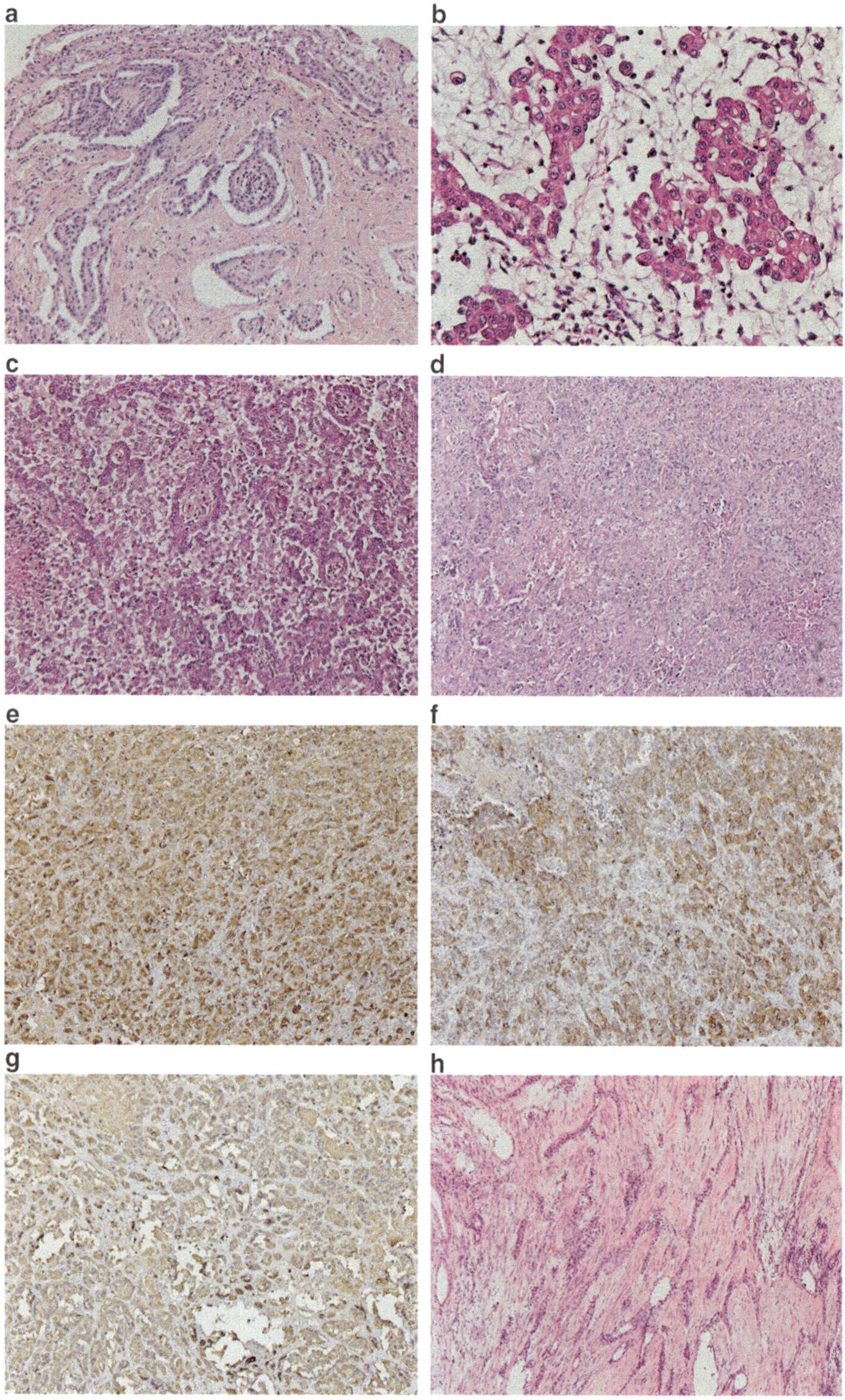

Fig. 2.1 Histopathology of mesothelial lesions and pseudomyxoma peritonei: (**a**) tubule-papillary type of diffuse malignant mesothelioma, HE, x200; (**b**) cytological features of diffuse malignant

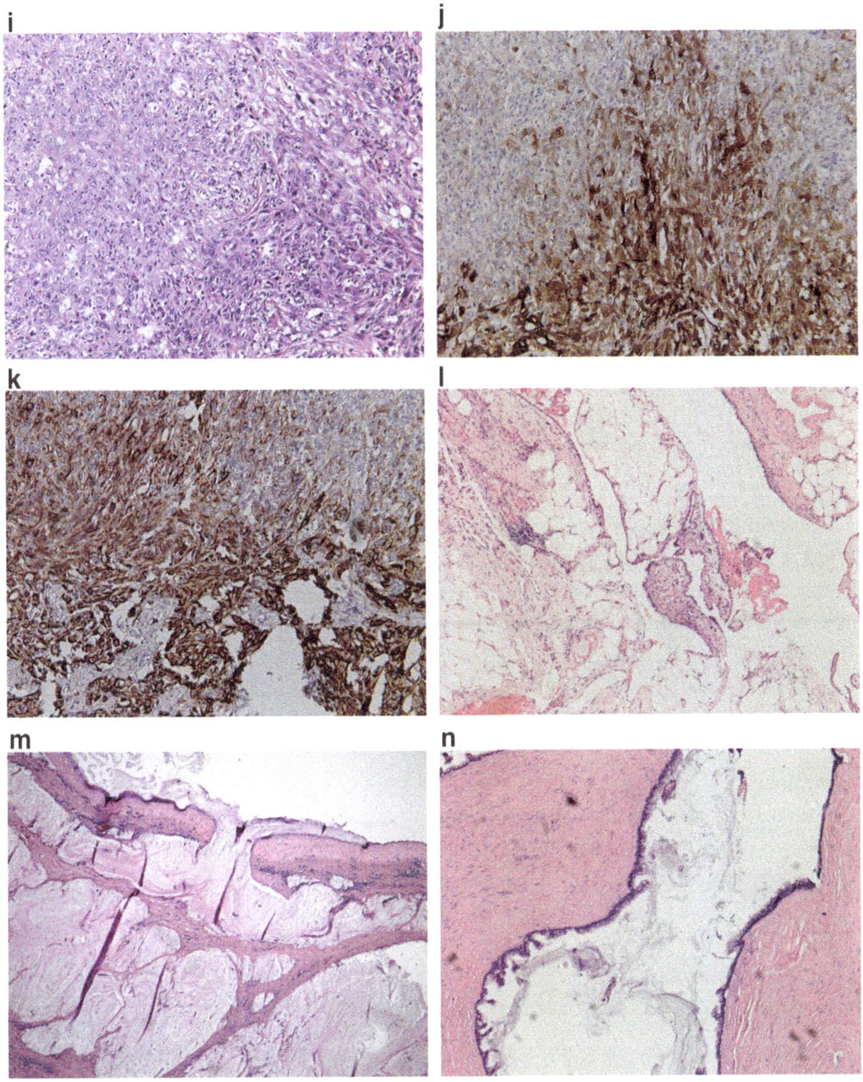

Fig. 2.1 (continued) mesothelioma, HE, x400; (**c**) papillary and trabecular growth pattern of diffuse malignant mesothelioma, HE, x200; (**d**) solid type of epithelioid malignant mesothelioma, HE, x200; (**e**) solid type of epithelioid malignant mesothelioma, immunohistochemical expression of calretinin, x200; (**f**) solid type of epithelioid malignant mesothelioma, immunohistochemical expression of CK5/6, x200; (**g**) solid type of epithelioid malignant mesothelioma, immunohistochemical expression of CK7, x200; (**h**) hypocellular biphasic malignant mesothelioma, HE, x100; (**i**) hypercellular admixture of highly atypical epithelioid and spindle cells of biphasic malignant mesothelioma, HE, x100; (**j**) biphasic malignant mesothelioma, immunohistochemical expression of calretinin, x100; (**k**) biphasic malignant mesothelioma, immunohistochemical expression of CK7, x100; (**l**) foci of reactive mesothelial proliferation near bulk of malignant mesothelioma, HE, x40; (**m**) accidental microscopic finding - dissected by mucin pools appendiceal wall with spreading of hypocellular mucinous tumour on serosal lining (low grade pseudomyxoma peritonei) , HE, x40; (**n**) single layer of bland appearing mucinous epithelium of low grade pseudomyxoma peritonei, HE, x100.

Histopathology WDPM is represented by well-differentiated papillary structures lined with a single layer of the flattened and/or cuboidal cells with centrally located nuclei and almost imperceptible nucleoli. The stroma of the tumor is paucicellular and often edematous. The nuclei of tumor cells are small, with smooth contours, and corresponds to a minimal atypia. WDPM has no or minimal mitotic activity [5].

The tumor cells form solid nests, tubular structures or cords in the fibrous stroma. In rare cases, WDPM can demonstrate features of adenomatoid tumor. Multinucleate giant cells can be found in stroma of WDPM.

Unlike malignant mesothelioma, WDPM has no widespread and deep invasions of surrounding tissues. At the same time, minimal surface invasion can be rarely detected in WDPM, which should be noted in the histological description. The presence in the tumor of psammoma bodies does not have any influence on the diagnosis.

Differential Diagnosis In the presence of nuclear atypia exceeding the minimal level, complex papillar architecture, presence of solid fields and invasion, the neoplasm should be regarded as malignant mesothelioma (if there are signs of mesothelial differentiation) or as high-grade serous carcinoma (there are no signs of mesothelial differentiation). Larger nodes (usually more than 2 cm) also suggest diagnosis of malignant mesothelioma. In difficult cases, immunohistochemistry with a panel of mesothelial and non-mesothelial antibodies is recommended.

Prognosis WDPM refers to borderline tumors, after its complete removal, the prognosis is favorable; after non-radical surgery, the disease relapses.

2.1.1.3 Diffuse Malignant Mesothelioma

Definition Malignant tumor of mesothelial origin, presenting with one of three histopathological subtypes: epithelioid, biphasic or sarcomatoid types.

Etiology Unlike the pleural analogue, the association of peritoneal mesotheliomogenesis with asbestos exposure has not been confirmed.

Clinical Features Clinical manifestations of diffuse malignant peritoneal mesothelioma are not specific and are not distinguishable from primary serous peritoneal, ovarian/tubal carcinoma with peritoneal dissemination or any other carcinomatosis. Most patients admit abdominal enlargement (presence of ascites) and pronounced abdominal discomfort at the time of examination. In rare cases the tumor can be diagnosed during surgical exploration or laparotomy performed for other reasons.

Gross Pathology In contrast to often accidentally detected small foci of AT or WDPM, MM is characterized by the presence of large merging thickened plaques and nodes on the parietal and visceral peritoneum with local formation of bosselated masses notably in major omentum. However, this picture is not specific and can be observed in primary peritoneal or metastatic ovarian serous carcinoma.

Cyto- And Histopathology During cytological examination of ascitic effusion specimens epithelioid MM cells are almost always found, whereas the frequency of sarcomatoid MM tumor cells detection is extremely small because the spindle cells of MM almost always do not peel off into the effusion fluid. In cytological specimens MM cells can demonstrate strips, clusters, morulae and papillary structures [8]. It is possible to detect psammoma bodies in cytological slides. Although the MM cells morphology can vary significantly from deceptively benign to polymorphic and malignant, they do not often have the degree of atypia that one can define in primary or metastatic peritoneal carcinoma [5]. At the same time, reactive mesothelium often shows signs (increased cellularity, nuclear polymorphism, mitotic activity) of overt malignancy. In these circumstances in a number of cases it is impossible to differentiate the reactive and neoplastic mesothelium in the cytological specimen. Moreover, cytology cannot reliably reveal the presence of invasion. The accuracy of the cytological diagnosis of MM remains low and according to several studies does not exceed 35% [9–11].

Based on its pathological features, peritoneal MM, like the pleural analogue, is divided into 3 main variants: epithelioid, biphasic and sarcomatoid. The incidence of these three types of tumors declines in the following order: epithelioid mesothelioma – biphasic mesothelioma – sarcomatoid mesothelioma. As mentioned above, histological and immunophenotypic features of MM of pleura, pericardium, peritoneum, and tunica vaginalis of the testicle are indistinguishable, which determines the absence of differential diagnostic criteria for MM of different anatomical localization.

Among all histologic variants of MM, the epithelioid MM is characterized by maximum variability of its histopathological growth patterns; moreover, often epithelioid MM may appear deceptively benign. It is not infrequent to appreciate the different histological patterns in the same tumor. In such cases, the tumor demonstrates a common combination of solid, tubulo-papillary and trabecular growth patterns; less often there can be found micropapillary, adenomatoid (microcystic), clear cell, transitional, deciduoid, signet-ring-cell and small cell patterns [8–10]. Common presence of psammoma bodies in the tumor tissue has no any diagnostic or prognostic significance [11]. The neoplastic stroma can vary from abundant to meager, with variable cytology (ranging from the hyalinized and almost acellular to hypercellular, which sometimes makes it difficult to differentiate epitheliod MM with the sarcomatoid component of biphasic MM). In 5–10% of cases, the stroma has myxoid changes (myxomatosis is caused by the accumulation of hyaluronic acid). As a rule, the mitotic activity of MM is low. Tumor cells are characterized by a mild or abundant eosinophilic cytoplasm, vesicular nuclei of benign appearance, and distinct cell membranes [8]. As tumor differentiation decreases, nuclear polymorphism and mitotic activity increases significantly. Different histopathological patterns on epithelioid MM are described below.

Tubulo-papillary variant is one of the most frequent patterns. It is well distinguished cytologically by marked features of mesothelial differentiation of the lesional cells, as well as by a variable combination of tubular and papillary structures lined with cuboidal benign-appearing cells or larger atypical ones surrounded by fibrotic stroma [8–11]. As usual this variant of epithelioid MM does not present any difficulties for diagnosis.

Trabecular variant is also a frequent growth pattern of epithelioid MM. Cytologically, it is readily demonstrates recognizable features of mesothelial differentiation. Histological appearance of trabecular MM presents with short and thin strands of relatively small cells imbedded in the stroma [9–11]. Like tubulo-papillary, trabecular MM presents no difficulties for diagnosis.

Micropapillary MM is relatively rare as a single form, but it can present as a minor component of otherwise typical epithelioid MM [8]. Micropapillary MM is histologically characterized by the presence of small papillary projections with no fibro-vascular cores [9, 10]. Micropapillary MM also presents no difficulties for diagnostics.

Adenomatoid variant is relatively rare as a single form of epithelioid MM [8]. Histologically, this adenomatoid pattern displays appearance of complex microcystic lace-like cellular structures [9, 10]. Due to the specificity of its growth pattern this variant of MM can be misdiagnosed as metastasis of adenocarcinoma or primary peritoneal cancer. Adenomatoid MM should be differentiated from another histologically similar, but benign mesothelial neoplasm – adenomatoid tumor.

Solid growth pattern can present the whole tumor bulk or be the one of its components [9–11]. Histologically, solid MM forms monotonous solid fields of epithelioid cells with abundant cytoplasm, dispersed or vesicular chromatin and distinct plasma membranes. Solid MM can be either easily recognized by routine light-microscopy [8], or cause diagnostic difficulties especially in presence of severe nuclear atypia, resembling large cell carcinoma or large cell lymphoma.

Lymphohistiocytoid epithelioid MM is rare and characterized by presence of dense lymphoid and histiocytoid infiltration intimately mixed with MM cells (similar to lymphoepithelioma-like carcinoma) [8]. In some cases inflammatory infiltrate can disguise lesional cells, giving the deceptive impression of a lymphoproliferative disease.

Clear-cell MM cannot be differentiated with metastatic clear-cell lung carcinoma or clear-cell renal cancer in most cases, and therefore requires immunohistochemistry for verification of the diagnosis.

Deciduoid growth pattern is a one of the rarest and not infrequently can be found in young women during or after pregnancy. It is far less common in male patients, as well as growth pattern of pleural MM [6, 12]. Tumor cells of deciduoid type have typical abundant vitreous cytoplasm resembling ectopic decidua on light microscopy. However, they differ from normal decidua by distinct nucleoli, high mitotic activity, immunohistochemical expression of cytokeratins and typical ultrastructural features.

Small cell MM has no such microscopic features of small cell lung cancer as impregnation of blood vessel wall by the basophilic nuclear material (Azzopardi phenomenon), nuclear molding and karyorrhexis. However, in most cases immunohistochemistry is required to clarify the diagnosis of small cell malignant mesothelioma.

Pleomorphic epithelioid MM is characterized by pronounced cellular and nuclear polymorphism and presents with patternless admixture of overtly malignant bizarre epithelioid, poligonal, spindle and multinucleated cells with scant or abundant cytoplasm and hyperchromatic nuclei. Pleomorphic MM demonstrates loss of any features of differentiation on light microscopy creating the appearance of sarcomatoid carcinoma of pleomorphic sarcoma and requires immunohistochemistry for diagnosis [13].

Sarcomatoid MM is the rarest one, it is characterized by proliferation of spindle-shaped cells forming multidirectional bundles of variable length or growing in patternless fashion. Cytologically, from case to case cells of sarcomatoid MM can differ significantly – from enlarged fusiform cells with abundant cytoplasm to thin fibroblast-like cells with scant cytoplasm [14]. Cellular and nuclear atypia, and mitotic activity vary in a similar way. Identification of heterogenous elements (neoplastic osteoid, chondroid, rhabdomyoblastic differentiation) in sarcomatoid MM has no prognostic significance. However, in such cases, it is necessary to differentiate that from skeletal and extraossal osteosarcomas or chondrosarcomas [11]. It is also necessary to differentiate the neoplastic bone or cartilage from intratumoral bone or chondroid metasplasia. An immunohistochemistry is necessary to exclude special types or undifferentiated pleomorphic sarcoma, reactive organizing serositis, and metastatic sarcomatoid carcinoma.

Desmoplastic MM is a subtype of sarcomatoid mesothelioma, which demonstrates a pronounced collagenous (desmoplastic) stroma and a low cellularity compared with other histological variants of MM. Histologically, the tumor is characterized by atypical cells with hyperchromatic nuclei sparsely distributed in the abundant dense collagenous stroma [14]. An important diagnostic feature is the proportion of acellular stroma accounting for not less than 50% of the tumor. Due to low cellularity and deceptively bland appearance in some cases it is ultimately important to differentiate desmoplastic MM with chronic organizing serositis. The main criteria of malignancy are the invasive growth into the underlying fat or the wall of the affected organ (IHC detection of CK-positive cells in adipose tissue), foci of necrosis, formation of cellular nodules. Prognosis for desmoplastic MM is similar to sarcomatoid mesothelioma [11].

Biphasic MM has no unique histological features and presents a combination of epithelioid and sarcomatoid growth patterns independent of their histological structures. The basic requirement for the histological diagnosis of "biphasic malignant mesothelioma" is the proportion of any tumor component (sarcomatoid or epithelioid) accounting for not less than 10% of the total tumor volume [8, 11].

Immunohistochemical Features Malignant mesothelioma demonstrate stable expression of panCK (AE1/AE3) and CK18 (sensitivity is 95%, specificity is 90–95%), calretinin (sensitivity is 99%, specificity is 90–95%), CK5/6 (sensitivity is 75–100% specificity is 80–90%), WT-1 (sensitivity is 70–95%, specificity is 98%), D2-40 (sensitivity is 90–100%, specificity is 85%) [11, 15–17]. The tumor cells also express GATA3 (50%) creating diagnostic difficulties for differentiation MM from breast cancer. The MM cells lack expression of vascular (CD31, CD34,

ERG), melanosomal (HMB45, Melan A, SOX-10) and hematological (CD20 and CD45) markers. About 5–10% of sarcomatoid mesotheliomas are keratin-negative, only 30% of these tumors express caltetinin, but more often the cells are D2-40-positive, rarely express CK5/6, WT-1, and mesothelin [11, 13, 18]. Some sarcomatoid MM demonstrate focal expression of vimentin, SMA, S-100 protein and desmin, which can lead to a diagnostic error if the results of the immunohistochemistry are incorrectly interpreted [18, 19]. Myogenin and Myo-D1 can be used for detection of heterologous rhabdomyoblastic component in biphasic or sarcomatoid MM. In terms of the correct diagnosis, it is necessary to keep in mind that rare cells of the peritoneal MM have a focal expression of non-mesothelial markers such as BerEP4 (7%), CD15 (4%), CEA (5%), ER (2%), PR (7%), and PAX-8 (6%) [20].

A comprehensive review of the differential diagnostic markers used in practical pathology was published by Ordonez [21]. The author describes most effective panels for the diagnosis of epithelioid MM – MM vs. serous carcinoma: MOC31, BerEP4, ER, PAX8, and calretinin; MM vs. renal cell carcinoma – D2-40, CK5/6, mesothelin, WT-1, CD15, PAX2, PAX8, RCC, and calretinin; MM vs. metastatic breast cancer – mesothelin, D2-40, MOC31, BerEP4, mammoglobin, GCDFP-15, calretinin, CK5/6, ER and PR (it should be keeping in mind that calretinin and CK5/6 can be expressed in basal-like triple negative breast cancer); MM vs. squamous cell carcinoma – D2-40, mesothelin, WT-1, MOC31, CEA, p63, and p40.

Although immunohistochemistry is widely used for verification of mesothelial differentiation of neoplastic cells, it should be noted that to date, there are no immunohistochemical markers that can effectively differentiate benign (reactive) mesotheliocytes from malignant ones.

Differential Diagnosis The most important diagnostic criterion of MM is invasion into the underlying tissues (fat tissue of the abdominal wall, major omentum, internal organs). In some cases, foci of invasive growth of MM can be minimal and not associated with desmoplastic reaction [1, 2]. However, microscopic evaluation of invasive growth can be difficult or even impossible in the small biopsies.

Potential diagnostic pitfall may occur as a result of incorrect interpretation of reactive mesothelial cells entrapped in masses of organizing fibrin on the surface of chronically inflamed serous cover or between lobules of fat [7]. In some cases of diffuse or localized *organized peritonitis*, one may encounter such a phenomenon as “fake fat”, an artificial change in the fibrin masses and connective tissue accompanying with the formation of rounded optically clear structures (vacuole-like spaces) similar to lipid drops of mature lipocytes. These artificial structures and true fat cells can be differentiated immunohistochemically: “fake fat” does not demonstrate expression of S100 protein, laminin and type IV collagen, and CK-positive entrapped mesothelial cells are located horizontally in relation to the serosal surface, and do not show vertically oriented growth like invasive MM cells.

In contrast to sarcomatoid MM, the organizing peritonitis has the following typical features: lack of CK-positive spindle cells in adipose tissue, histological storiform grown pattern, vertically oriented to the surface of the peritoneum capillaries, uniform thickness of cell proliferation without nodal thickenings, “zonation” (gradual decrease of cellularity descending away from the peritoneal surface). Necrotic foci and inflammatory infiltration are not informative for differential diagnosis [1, 2, 22].

WDPM has no cellular stratification, complex papillary architecture and mixed cell populations, which are typical for low grade serous tumors; it neither has high mitotic activity and pronounced atypia, which is typical for high grade serous carcinoma. The latter makes it possible to distinguish the WDPM from MM. Absence of abdominal surgery in the anamnesis or inflammatory processes of peritoneum, as well as formation of true papillae allow to differentiate WDPM from reactive mesothelial hyperplasia [5, 7].

Another peritoneal lesion that in some cases requires differential diagnosis from MM is the *multicystic mesothelioma* (peritoneal inclusion cyst).

Solitary fibrous tumor (SFT) of the peritoneum does not demonstrate macroscopic diffuse growth pattern typical for MM, but usually forms a single mass. SFT cells are positive for CD34, STAT6, bcl-2, and negative for cytokeratin and mesothelial markers [11, 23].

Sarcomatoid carcinoma is characterized by cytokeratin expression and lack of mesothelial differentiation markers [11].

Undifferentiated pleomorphic sarcoma demonstrates vimentin expression, in the absence of keratins and mesothelial markers [11].

Reactive mesothelial hyperplasia does not have high cellularity in the stromal part of the lesion and is characterized by zonation, but it can also have pronounced cellular atypia and small foci of necrosis [24]. In some cases if microscopic examination demonstrates a massive solid tumor with microscopic features of MM, detection of invasive growth becomes unnecessary for diagnosis [1, 2].

Due to its macroscopic and microscopic growth patterns, MM can be misinterpreted as secondary or primary peritoneal *serous carcinoma*. In contrast to MM, primary or metastatic high grade serous carcinoma forms more complex papillary structures, sometimes protruding into the lumen, as well as more pronounced cytological atypia. Since psammoma bodies can be found not only in serous carcinoma, their presence isn't useful for differential diagnostics. Acidic mucins (hyaluronic acid) easily detected on histochemically stained slides are characteristic for MM, whereas neutral mucins are typical for metastatic carcinoma. Synchronous expression of vimentin, thrombomodulin, calretinin, h-caldesmon, D2-40 and CK in the absence of CEA, B72.3, CD15 and BerEP4 expression in tumor cells are typical for MM. Serous carcinoma, regardless of organ origin, is characterized by a directly opposite immunophenotype [25, 26].

Homozygous p16 deletion, determined by FISH, and loss of immunohistochemical expression of BAP1 (not in all cases) are relatively specific MM molecular biomarkers. The two above-mentioned markers are the most effective for MM diagnosis. It was found that the loss of BAP1 expression is also heterogeneous in different MM variants: loss of BAP1 expression is rarely found in sarcomatoid and desmoplastic MM [1, 2].

It should be noted that to date, there are no specific mesothelioma markers. This fact makes it necessary to consider not only immunohistochemical and light-optical features, but also take into account clinical and radiological data for diagnosis of malignant mesothelioma.

Prognosis As with pleural analogue there are two most informative and independent prognostic factors for peritoneal MM: tumor stage according to TNM Classification and histopathological type of MM. Despite the high mortality of the patients the highest survival rate was observed in patients with epithelioid type of MM, gradually decreasing in patients with biphasic variant and being minimal for sarcomatoid MM.

2.1.1.4 Prognostic Parameters of Malignant Peritoneal Mesothelioma.

Cerutto et al. proposed a method for prognostic stratification of patients with epithelioid malignant mesothelioma based on the account of nuclear atypia and nucleolar characteristics – Table 2.2.

Table 2.2 Nuclear-nucleolar grading of malignant peritoneal epithelioid mesothelioma

Method requirements	Only predominating in current tumor sample nuclear size of neoplastic cells is taken into account (using micrometer scale bar or erythrocyte/small lymphocyte).		
	In presence of intratumoral heterogeneity of nuclear diameter, only nuclei with largest diameter are taken into account.		
	In presence in tumor sample of rare or scarcely distributed neoplastic cells with more pleomorphic nuclei than in predominating population these rare cells are not taking into account [modified from Cerutto et al].		
Prognostic group	**Range, μ**	**Nuclei**	**Nucleoli**
Group 1	< 20	Neoplastic nuclei looks «absolutely the same», i.e. monomorphic small, round, with homogeneous dark chromatin, and diameter no more than 1-1,3 diameter of erythrocyte	Small, rare, indiscernible in most nuclei
Group 2	20–30	Nuclei are «still the same» – round, slightly enlarged, with cleared granulated chromatin, and diameter no more than 1,5-2 diameter of erythrocyte	Well discernible in most nuclei, with diameter less than 3 μ
Group 3	30–40	Nuclei «are not the same anymore» – discernible variation of nuclear diameter, eccentric clearing of chromatin, nuclear diameter equals 3-5 diameter of erythrocyte	Well discernible, with diameter 3 to 5 μ
Group 4	> 40	Nuclei are extremely polymorphous – striking variation of nuclear diameter with eccentric clearing of chromatin (large, vesicular and bizarre nuclei), nuclear diameter more than 6 diameter of erythrocyte	Well discernible, large, with diameter 6 μ and more

2.2 Non-neoplastic Mesothelial Lesions

2.2.1 Reactive Mesothelial Hyperplasia

Definition benign non-neoplastic proliferation of mesothelium.

Etiology RMH is often found during microscopic studies as single or multiple foci of proliferation of peritoneum near adnexa in chronic salpingitis or endometriosis as a stereotypic reaction on chronic inflammation and/or effusion in peritoneal cavity; in greater omentum near the metastases of ovarian cancer; in a wall of hernial sac or at the site of previous laparoscopy [24, 26]. Distinguishing RMH from malignant mesothelioma may be difficult in some cases, especially with small biopsies, which may cause diagnostic errors.

Histopathology RMH can have highly variable structures including solid, trabecular, tubular, papillary and tubulo-papillary patterns of growth. The lesion can be surrounded by fibrous tissue or organizing masses of fibrin. Of note, foci of RMH are limited by serous membrane with a gradual or sometimes abrupt transition between normal and hyperplastic mesothelium [24]. On cytological specimens, reactive mesothelial cells can demonstrate nuclear atypia (ranging from moderate to severe) and cytoplasmic vacuoles with acidic mucins, less frequently significant clearing of cytoplasm can be appreciated. In rare cases, psammoma bodies and rhabdomyoblast-like mesothelial cells are found [26]. Diffuse inflammatory infiltrate, CD68-positive histiocytes, siderophages and reactive angiomatosis are often present at foci of RMH [24].

The following histologic features of RMH may potentially mislead to a false positive diagnosis of malignant mesothelioma: high cellularity, increased mitotic activity, foci of necrosis, entrapment of single reactive mesothelial cells or even cell clusters in organizing fibrinous effusion imitating invasion.

Differential Diagnostics Differential diagnosis spectrum of RMH is highly variable and includes MM, metastatic cancer, and serous borderline or malignant ovarian tumors.

In contrast to MM, RMH foci do not form macroscopically distinguishable nodes on peritoneal surface. The cells do not have large cytoplasmic vacuoles. There are no significant signs of the subjacent tissue invasion. The full spectrum of diagnostic criteria for RMH is listed in Table 2.3.

According to recent studies it is well established that some immunohistochemical markers as EMA, GLUT-1, IMP-3, and p53 are ineffective in differentiation of MM and RMH [1, 2, 26]. In particular, the immunohistochemical markers were shown to distinguish the malignant and benign mesothelial lesions, but exclusively from the statistic point of view [1, 2]. Therefore, abovementioned markers aren't applicable for an analysis of individual cases. Analysis of proliferative activity of reactive and neoplastic cells also reveals an overlapping between both reactive and neoplastic

Table 2.3 Differential diagnostics of RMH and MM

	Reactive mesothelial hyperplasia	Malignant mesothelioma
Basic criteria		
Stromal invasion	Absent	Present
Cells	Cells are limited by pleura surface	High numbers of cells with stromal reaction
Papillary structures	Simple, one layer	Complex, with cell stratification
Growth type	Superficial	Expansive nodules with complex architecture
Zonation of the lesion	Decreasing of lesional cell density with depth	Absent
Blood vessels	Capillaries are located perpendicularly the serosal surface	Capillaries are located unevenly
Secondary criteria		
Cellular atypia	Limited by the area of an organizing exudate on inflamed serosa	In any part of the lesion
Necrosis	Possible	Possible
Mitotic activity	Mitoses may be present	There are often few mitoses, but some of them can be are atypical

lesions [24]. Another molecular marker expressed exclusively in reactive mesothelium is desmin [26]. A diffuse and intensive expression of calretinin, desmin, CD44 alongside with absence of E-cadherin in most of the cases allows distinguishing between reactive mesothelium and primary or metastatic peritoneum cancer. Despite published results it is not recommended to use any immunohistochemical stains except keratin antibodies in differentiation of benign and malignant mesothelium.

Prognosis Prognosis of reactive mesothelial hyperplasia is favorable.

2.2.2 *Multicystic Mesothelioma*

Definition non-neoplastic benign polycystic lesion of peritoneal mesothelium.

Synonym peritoneal cystic mesothelioma.

Etiology, Epidemiology In contrast to malignant mesothelioma, MCM is prevalent in young and middle-aged women, and like MM, it is not associated with carcinogenic influence of asbestos.

Clinical and Morphological Features MCM is diffusely spreading on abdominal peritoneum without signs of invasion, forming multiple thin-walled cysts with a semitransparent fluid [5]. MCM predominantly affects peritoneum lining abdominal wall and pelvic visceral lining. In few cases MCM can produce large amounts of colloid masses on peritoneal surface grossly imitating pseudomyxoma peritonei. In contrast to malignant mesothelioma, MCM do not form macroscopically distinguishable plaque-like foci with necrotic sites on peritoneal surface and do not demonstrate prominent cellular atypia.

Histopathology Inner surface of fibrous cystic walls is lined by one layer of cytologically benign flattened cells without stratification or formation of papillary structures [1, 2].

Differential Diagnostics In some cases cystic lymphangioma may imitate MCM. However, cystic lymphangioma is more frequently encountered in children and male teenagers. Lymphangioma is often localized outside pelvic cavity within mesentery of small intestine, colon, greater omentum or in retroperitoneal space. The lymphoangioma cysts frequently contains chylous fluid; lymphoid clusters and smooth muscle cells may be present in mural sites of lymphangioma [26]. In contrast to lymphoangioma, MCM cells do not express podoplanin (D2-40) and are keratin-positive [7].

Prognosis MCM prognosis is favorable. The disease might be recurrent if a lesion is not totally resected by the surgeon.

2.3 Selected Metastatic Peritoneal Lesions

2.3.1 Peritoneal Pseudomyxoma

Definition Peritoneal pseudomyxoma (PP) has its special place among a wide group of secondary peritoneal neoplastic lesions. Being a historic descriptive clinical term, PP is used by clinicians for description of large amounts of mucinous agglomerates fixed on serous peritoneal surface. Being an uninformative descriptive diagnosis it requires identification of a primary anatomic location of neoplastic process and histological grade of the tumor [27].

Synonyms low-grade PP – disseminated peritoneal adenomucinosis; high-grade PP-mucinous carcinomatosis. Terms "mucinous borderline tumor" and "well differentiated mucinous adenocarcinoma" are not recommended.

Origin of Tumor Well-differentiated mucinous low-grade tumors are often may cause accumulation of mucin in the abdominal cavity. Vast majority of these tumors has appendiceal origin. Thus, if PP is detected, appendectomy with a subsequent total pathological examination of appendix is necessary.

Mucinous tumors of colon, pancreas, urachus, gallbladder and stomach cause PP much rarer [28]. Despite an initial opinion, mucinous ovarian tumors, including borderline, may lead to PP very infrequently, except for mucinous adenocarcinoma with intestinal or appendicular differentiation developed in mature teratoma [27, 29].

It should be stressed, that PP classification, which would describe all the clinical and pathological features of biology of these tumors, is currently absent. Carr et al. [27] suggested dividing pseudomyxoma peritonei into two main types: mucinous tumors of low malignant potential (G1) and mucinous adenocarcinomas of high malignant potential, including moderately and poorly differentiated mucinous adenocarcinoma (G2-G3) and signet-ring cell carcinoma (G3). Table 2.4 presents WHO classification of pseudomyxoma peritonei [28].

Gross Pathology Characteristic peritoneal pattern of dissemination of PP is noted. It is well established that PP frequently "avoids" serous lining of small intestine, preferring greater omentum, right dome of diaphragm, right retrohepatic space, ligament of Treitz, right flank and pelvic cavity [27]. The tumor invasion into ovaries may be present as double-sided lesions (more frequent) or as isolated dissemination of right ovary [29]. Macroscopically, the ovaries are dramatically increased in size and deformed by single or multiple cysts with a semitransparent mucinous fluid.

Histopathology Microscopic examination reveals large mucinous pools with rare floating mucous-containing neoplastic cells. In case of ovarian involvement, an dissection of gonadal stroma by mucinous pools is noted («ovarian pseudomyxoma») [29]. Another special feature of low-grade PP is absence of invasion into subserous tissues or affected organs which is typical for other malignant tumors. On the other hand, high-grade mucinous tumors usually demonstrate wide spread invasive growth.

Low-grade PP may be presented both by single cells and by small clusters, strips of columnal mucinous epithelium and gland-like structures, which are located peripherally or float in mucous lakes and contain appreciable quantities of mucin in the cytoplasm. Cellular atypia, as a rule, is minimal, which is typical for well-differentiated low-grade appendiceal tumors. If signet ring cellular cells are noted, the tumor should be considered as a high-grade adenocarcinoma [27].

Table 2.4 Classification of peritoneal pseudomyxoma

Grade of malignancy	Histologic pattern	Cytological features	Contents of mucin in cells	Mitotic activity
Low	Scant strips or small clusters of cells floating within abundant pools of mucin, without signs of invasive growth	Tumor cells may be deceptively bland. Small nuclei with minimal atypia	On the whole, variable. Signet ring cells are absent.	Low or absent
High	Numerous strips of cells, cribriform structures or clusters of tumor cells floating in abundant mucin; vast invasion of subjacent tissues is observed	At least focally prominent atypia	Variable. Signet ring cells may appear.	Frequent, including atypical

It must be stressed that morphological diagnosis of PP is rather hard, as mucin deposits significantly prevail over tumor cells, thus, their detection requires extensive sampling.

Mucinous carcinomatosis is another “face” of PP caused by high-grade adenocarcinoma, originating from different organs of abdominal cavity. A characteristic feature of this group is a typical for most of carcinomas infiltrating growth, severe cellular and nuclear atypia, frequent lymph node metastases or distant metastases.

Metastatic Spread Lymphogenous or distant metastases in low-grade PP are extremely rare. As a rule, such cases result from a more malignant mucinous tumor unrevealed during pathologic examination of surgical specimen [29].

Immunohistochemical Features Pseudomyxoma cells of appendicular origin typically possess intestinal phenotype (CK7-/CK20+), but in 30% of cases express CK7 that distinguishes them from similar tumors of colorectal origin. Besides, appendicular tumors, as well as colon mucinous adenocarcinoma express markers of epithelial (CK8, CK18, CK19) and intestinal differentiation (MUC2, CDX-2 и DPC4) [26]. More than 80% of appendicular mucinous adenocarcinomas, like the same tumors in stomach, pancreas and ovaries, express MUC5AC.

Moreover, similar phenotype (CK7+/CK20+) is present both in mucinous tumors of ovaries and appendix, which may cause significant difficulties in differential diagnostics of PP origin [30]. Thus, the most prolific panel includes the following markers: CK7, CK20, CDX2, MUC2 and MUC5AC (Table 2.5).

Lack of CK7 expression along with a diffuse and strong CK20 expression identifies colorectal origin of tumor; at the same time, phenotype CK7+/CK20- is more typical for primary mucinous ovarian tumors [15, 25, 30]. If the markers are expressed synchronously, it is critical to evaluate a distribution and intensity of staining. For example, a diffuse and strong expression CK7 with focal CK20 expression evidences the most probable gonadal origin of the tumor, but not the colorectal one and vice versa. Faint focal expression of CDX-2 is frequently observed in mucinous neoplasms of ovaries and pancreas, thus, allowing their discrimination from similar colorectal tumors, there its expression is diffuse and intense. Rare mucinous tumors developed within mature ovarian teratoma possess phenotype of lower gastrointestinal tract (CK7-/CK20+/CDX2+). Differential diagnostics of such cases relies solely on the analysis of clinicopathologic data with an obligatory exclusion of gastrointestinal tumor [15].

Signet-ring cell carcinoma may cause PP in several cases. If signet-ring cells are detected, it is recommended to determine tumor origin with following panel: CK7, CK20, CK5/6, TTF-1, CDX-2, MUC2, ER, PR [25, 31, 32].

Differential Diagnostics Spectrum of differential diagnosis of PP includes endometriosis with myxoid changes, myxoid leiomyosarcoma and aggressive angiomyxoma [27]. Despite the described rare cases of malignant progression of mucinous peritoneal tumor accompanied by decreasing of cell differentiation, vast

Table 2.5 Immunophenotype of peritoneal pseudomyxoma depending on tumor

Anatomic origin of mucinous tumor	CK7	CK20	MUC5AC	MUC2	CDX2	CDH-17	PAX-8[a]	Other stains
Appendix	35% Focal to diffuse	100%	80%	100%	100%	95%	0	
Colon	15%, Rare cells	90%	15–33%	55%	90%	95%	0	
Rectum	+	+			+	95%	0	
Ovary (intestinal type)	95%	40–65% focal	95%	15%	35% Focal to diffuse	ND	60%[b]	No expression of ER and PR
Ovary (cervical type)	+	0	ND	ND	0	ND	+	Frequent expression of ER, PR
Endocervix	ND	ND	0	0	ND	0	95%	P16+, HPV+
Pancreas	95%	40%	85%	5%	15% focal	ND	0	DPC4-
Stomach	50%	40%	80%	50%	20–90%[c]	90%	0	ND
Breast	90%	10% focal	0	0	0	0	0	GCDFP-15+, mammoglobin+, ER±, PR±, WT1-, CA125-

ND no data

[a]Only strong expression is considered positive. Polyclonal antibodies to PAX-8 cross-react with PAX5 and PAX6

[b]Expression is absent in mucinous tumors, originating from teratoma

[c]Expression is heterogeneous in diffuse type tumors and homogenously intense in intestinal tumors

majority of pseudomyxoma peritonei cases does not demonstrate invasive growth, and lymphogenic or hematogenic metastases [27].

Differential diagnosis of PP and primary mucinous ovarian tumors is presented in Table 2.6.

Prognosis Determination of tumor histologic type is necessary for the prognosis of planned treatment. Pathological report should include information about histologic type of tumor, grade, as well as tumor origin.

Conclusion It should be noted that the modern surgical pathology of primary and metastatic peritoneal tumors relies on meticulous analysis of clinical, radiological histopathological features of the lesion, as well as the use of additional diagnostics, including immunohistochemistry and molecular pathology, allowing verification of the diagnosis, clarification of the prognosis of the disease and the clinician to choose the most optimal patient management.

Table 2.6 Signs of differential diagnostics of PP and primary mucinous ovarian tumors

Pathological features	Pseudomyxoma peritonei affecting ovaries	Primary mucinous ovarian tumor
Ovary dimensions	Medium (7–16 cm)	Massive (18–22 cm)
Lesion localization	Two-sided – 80% cases	One-sided – 95% cases
Tumor localization	Ovarian surface, cortex, stroma	Frequently in stroma, in case of cystic rupture may spread onto ovarian surface
Presence of pseudomyxoma ovarii	Wide spread	Absent/localized
Amount of mucinous cells	Usually scarce	Abundant
Presence of mucinous tumor in appendix/other organs of gastrointestinal tract	Always	Never/occasional coincidence

References

1. Husain AN, Colby T, Ordonez N, Krausz T, Attanoos R, Beasley MB et al (2013) Guidelines for pathologic diagnosis of malignant mesothelioma: 2012 update of the consensus statement from the IMIG. Arch Pathol Lab Med 137(5):647–667
2. Husain AN, Colby TV, Ordonez NG, Allen TC, Attanoos RL et al (2018) Guidelines for pathologic diagnosis of malignant mesothelioma 2017 update of the consensus statement from the IMIG. Arch Pathol Lab Med 142(1):89–108
3. Alvorado-Cabrero I (2009) Pathology of the fallopian tube and broad ligament. In: Nucci MR, Oliva E (eds) Gynecologic pathology. Elsevier, Edinburgh/Churchill, pp 346–348
4. Daya D, Cheung ANY et al (2014) Mesothelial tumors. In: Kurman RJ, Carcangiu ML, Herrington S (eds) WHO classification of tumors of female reproductive organs. IARC, Lyon, pp 90–91
5. Levy AD, Arnaiz J, Shaw JC, Sobin LH (2008) From the archives of the AFIP: primary peritoneal tumors: imaging features with pathologic correlation. Radiographics 28(2):583–607
6. Colgan TJ, Chang MC (2011) Fallopian tube and peritoneum. In: Soslow RA, Tornos C (eds) Diagnostic pathology of ovarian tumors. Springer, New York, pp 267–275
7. Mok SC, Schorge JO, Weich WR et al (2003) Peritoneal tumors. In: Tavassoli FA, Devilee P (eds) WHO classification of tumors. Pathology & genetics of tumors of breast and female genital organs. IARC Press, Lyon, pp 197–202
8. Baker PM, Clement PB, Young RH (2005) Malignant peritoneal mesothelioma in women: a study of 75 cases with emphasis on their morphologic spectrum and differential diagnosis. Am J Clin Pathol 123(5):724–737
9. Henderson DW, Reid G, Kao SC, van Zandwijk N, Klebe S (2013) Challenges and controversies in the diagnosis of malignant mesothelioma: part 2. Malignant mesothelioma subtypes, pleural synovial sarcoma, molecular and prognostic aspects of mesothelioma, BAP1, aquaporin-1 and microRNA. J Clin Pathol 66(10):854–861
10. Henderson DW, Reid G, Kao SC, van Zandwijk N, Klebe S (2013) Challenges and controversies in the diagnosis of mesothelioma: part 1. Cytology-only diagnosis, biopsies, immunohistochemistry, discrimination between mesothelioma and reactive mesothelial hyperplasia, and biomarkers. J Clin Pathol 66(10):847–853
11. Travis WD, Brambilla E, Burke AP, Mrx A, Nicholson AG (2014) WHO classification of tumors of the kung, pleura, thymus and heart. IARC, Lyon
12. Ordonez NG (2012) Deciduoid mesothelioma: report of 21 cases with review of the literature. Mod Pathol 25(11):1481–1495

13. Ordonez NG (2012) Pleomorphic mesothelioma: report of 10 cases. Mod Pathol 25(7):1011–1022
14. Klebe S, Brownlee NA, Mahar A, Burchette JL, Sporn TA, Vollmer RT, Roggli VL (2010) Sarcomatoid mesothelioma: a clinical-pathologic correlation of 326 cases. Mod Pathol 23(3):470–479
15. Dabbs DJ (2010) Diagnostic immunohistochemistry: theranostic and genomic applications. Saunders, Philadelphia
16. Soomro IN, Oliveira R, Ronan J, Chaudry ZR, Johnson J (2005) Expression of mesothelial markers in malignant mesotheliomas: an immunohistochemical evaluation of 173 cases. J Pak Med Assoc 55(5):205–209
17. Suster S, Moran CA (2006) Applications and limitations of immunohistochemistry in the diagnosis of malignant mesothelioma. Adv Anat Pathol 13(6):316–329
18. Attanoos RL, Dojcinov SD, Webb R, Gibbs AR (2000) Anti-mesothelial markers in sarcomatoid mesothelioma and other spindle cell neoplasms. Histopathology 37(3):224–231
19. Lucas DR, Pass HI, Madan SK, Adsay NV, Wali A, Tabaczka P, Lonardo F (2003) Sarcomatoid mesothelioma and its histological mimics: a comparative immunohistochemical study. Histopathology 42(3):270–279
20. Tandon RT, Jimenez-Cortez Y, Taub R, Borczuk AC (2018) Immunohistochemistry in peritoneal mesothelioma: a single-center experience of 244 cases. Arch Pathol Lab Med 142(2):236–242
21. Ordonez NG (2013) Application of immunohistochemistry in the diagnosis of epithelioid mesothelioma: review and update. Hum Pathol 44:1–19
22. Mangano WE, Cagle PT, Churg A, Vollmer RT, Roggli VL (1998) The diagnosis of desmoplastic malignant mesothelioma and its distinction from fibrous pleurisy: a histologic and immunohistochemical analysis of 31 cases including p53 immunostaining. Am J Clin Pathol 110(2):191–199
23. Fletcher CDM, Bridge JA, Lee JC (2013) Extrapleural solitary fibrous tumor. In: Fletcher CDM, Bridge JA, Hogendoorn PCW, Mertens F (eds) WHO classification of tumors of soft tissue and bone. Lyon, IARC Press, pp 80–83
24. Weiss SW, Goldblum JR (2008) Enzinger and Weiss's soft tissue tumors, 5th edn. Mosby Elsevier, Philadelphia
25. Bahrami A, Luan DT, Jae YR (2008) Undifferentiated tumor: true identity by immunohistochemistry. Arch Pathol Lab Med 132:326–348
26. Clement PB, Young RH (2010) The peritoneum. In: Mills SE (ed) Sternberg's diagnostic surgical pathology, 5th edn. Lippincott Williams & Wilkins, Philadelphia, pp 2393–2412
27. Carr NJ, Emory TS, Sobin LH (2003) Epithelial neoplasms of the appendix. In: Odze RD, Goldblum RG (eds) Surgical pathology of the GI tract, liver, biliary tract and pancreas. IARC Press, Lyon, pp 645–647
28. Carr NJ, Sobin LH (2010) Adenocarcinoma of the appendix. In: Bosman FT, Carneiro F, Hruban RH et al (eds) WHO classification of tumors of the digestive system. IARC, Lyon, pp 122–124
29. Yemelyanova A, Seidman JD (2011) Metastatic tumors. In: Soslow RA, Tornos C (eds) Diagnostic pathology of ovarian tumors. Springer, New York, pp 140–143
30. Vang R, Ronnett BM (2009) Metastatic and miscellaneous tumors of the ovary. In: Nucci MR, Oliva E (eds) Gynecologic pathology. Elsevier, Philadelphia, pp 539–564
31. Terada T (2013) An immunohistochemical study of primary signet-ring cell carcinoma of the stomach and colorectum: expression of EMA, CEA, CA19–9, CDX-2, p53, Ki-67 antigen, TTF-1 and p63 in normal mucosa and in 42 cases. Int J Clin Exp Pathol 6(4):630–638
32. Terada T (2013) An immunohistochemical study of primary signet-ring cell carcinoma of the stomach and colorectum: cytokeratin profile in 42 cases. Int J Clin Exp Pathol 6(4):703–710

Chapter 3
Up to Date Approaches to Treatment of Patients with Pseudomyxoma Peritonei and Peritoneal Mesothelioma

Amir G. Abdulaev, Boris E. Polotskiy, and Mikhail M. Davydov

Abstract Pseudomyxoma peritonei and peritoneal mesothelioma are rare malignant diseases associated with poor prognosis. Cytoreductive surgery and intraoperative hyperthermic intraperitoneal chemotherapy have been used as locoregional treatment modes for patients with perithoneal mesothelioma. Combination of these methods allows increasing treatment efficiency of this cohort of cancer patients.

Keywords Peritoneal mesothelioma · Pseudomyxoma peritonei · Cytoreductive surgery · Intraperitoneal chemotherapy

3.1 Patient Examination

Regardless of the tumor dissemination grade, patients with pseudomyxoma and mesothelioma should undergo a standard examination including the following procedures.

1. Blood tests: general clinical test, biochemical, coagulogram, blood type, rhesus factor, tumor markers (in case of pseudomyxoma CEA, CA-19.9, CA-125, in case of mesothelioma CEA, CA15.3, CA-125).
2. X-ray examination of chest organs.
3. Ultrasound analysis of abdomen, cervical-supraclavicular areas, pelvis, lower limb veins.
4. CT/MRI of abdomen and pelvis with i.v. contrast, if no contraindications.
5. Esophageal gastro-duodenoscopy.

A. G. Abdulaev · B. E. Polotskiy (✉) · M. M. Davydov
Oncologist and Surgeon Thoracic Research Department, N.N. Blokhin National Medical Research Center, Moscow, Russia

© Springer Nature Switzerland AG 2019

M. V. Kiselevskiy et al. (eds.), *Malignant Mesothelioma and Pseudomyxoma*, https://doi.org/10.1007/978-3-319-99510-6_3

6. If there are indications (massive malignant lesions of pelvis and mesogastrium), colonoscopy and cystoscopy with catheterization of ureters should be performed prior to the surgery. The latter is considered important for prevention of iatrogenic intraoperative injury of the ureter. In case of compression and pain in the abdominal cavity, irrigoscopy and rectoromanoscopy are performed.

3.1.1 Assessment of Functional Status

Cytoreductive surgery as a stage therapy combined with intraperitoneal chemotherapy is a significant injury to the patient, and therefore, all patients should undergo ECG, advanced spirometry, echocardiography. In case of indications (CHD, arrhythmia), the patients undergo Holter monitoring, stress ECHO, myocardial scintigraphy or coronary angiography.

A thorough examination is necessary to answer two questions: (1) how much the disease is extended, and (2) whether the patient's status is good to tolerate well the planned extension of the treatment.

In complicated clinical situations, if a patient had a concomitant (competing) pathology, we held a consultation with participation of a resuscitator, therapist, anesthesiologist and surgeon, which allowed us to answer the second question with sufficient probability. However, at the first stage of the study, due to little experience, we faced a serious problem of assessing the real extention of the disease and operability, i.e. feasibility of performing optimal cytoreduction.

Besides classification P1-P3 (JGCA, 1998), we referred to PCI (peritoneal cancer index) to evaluate the disease extension with PCI being determined at intraoperational revision. In addition, we took into consideration the lesion size (LS, or Lesion size), and localization of tumor dissemination in the peritoneum divided into 13 areas.

Maximal lesion size is determined for every area (LS 0–3), and peritoneal cancer index is calculated as a result of summarizing them. PCI was estimated only in the study patients' group (Table 3.1).

We divided cancer peritoneal index values into the intervals 1–5, 5–10, 10–15 and over 15 for a more appropriate analysis.

In our opinion, the use of this classification has revealed a number of significant drawbacks, which on the whole, limit its feasibility for widespread use and planning of surgical intervention in pseudomyxoma and mesothelioma.

Table 3.1 The degree of intraperitoneal dissemination in the studied patients with pseudomyxoma: P1-P3, PCI

Grade of i/p dissemination P1-P3	Grade of i/p dissemination PCI
P1, n = 6	1–5, n = 6
P2, n = 10	1–5, n = 4
	5–10, n = 4
	10–15, n = 2
P3, n = 27	10–15, n = 19
	15, n = 8
Total n = 43	

Evaluation of tumor operability, i.e. the possibility of performing optimal cytoreductive surgery according to CT data is ambiguous. Thus, it is possible to highlight indirect radiological signs which indicate inoperable status (Figs. 3.1, 3.2 and 3.3).

On the other hand, unclear CT signs of the disease and, accordingly, low PCI in some cases also resulted in appropriate tumor removal (Figs. 3.4, 3.5 and Fig. 3.6). However, we should mention that those were always recurrences, where interventions were performed repeatedly.

In general, a typical CT-sign of pseudomyxoma was the diffuse peritoneal lesion because of cystic solid lesions (Fig. 3.6). Malignant lesions often localize on the peritoneum of the diaphragm domes, in the large omentum, and small pelvis. At the same time, we made correction of planning volume of surgical intervention in all observations taking into account intraoperative revision.

In rare cases, CT revealed signs of malignant lesions of the appendix, and mucocele with calcified capsule could develop, which is clearly seen in the pictures (Fig. 3.7).

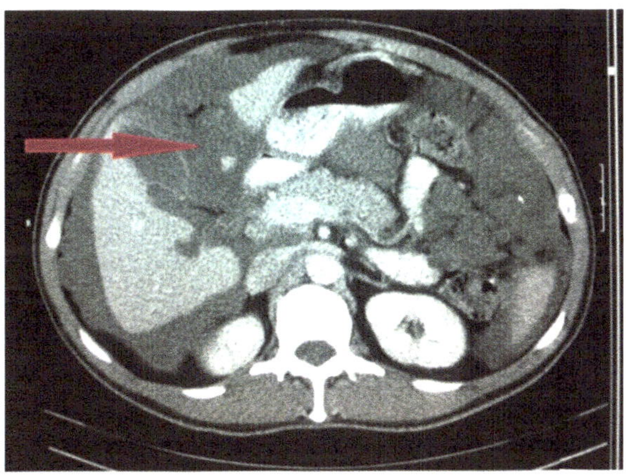

Fig. 3.1 Affected capsule of the liver with compression of its parenchyma. CT sign

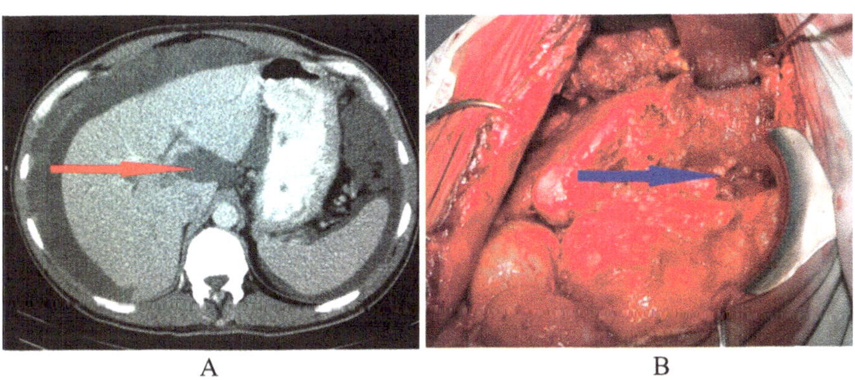

Fig. 3.2 Infiltration of hepato-duodenal and falciform ligaments. (**a**) CT sign; (**b**) Step of surgery

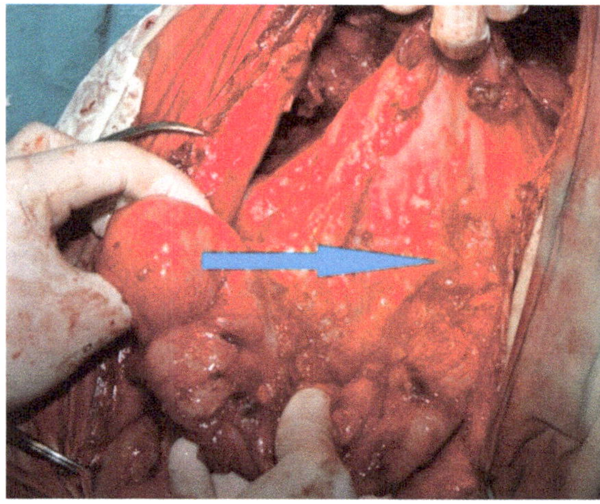

Fig. 3.3 Tumor bulk in the area of the omental bursa. Step of surgery

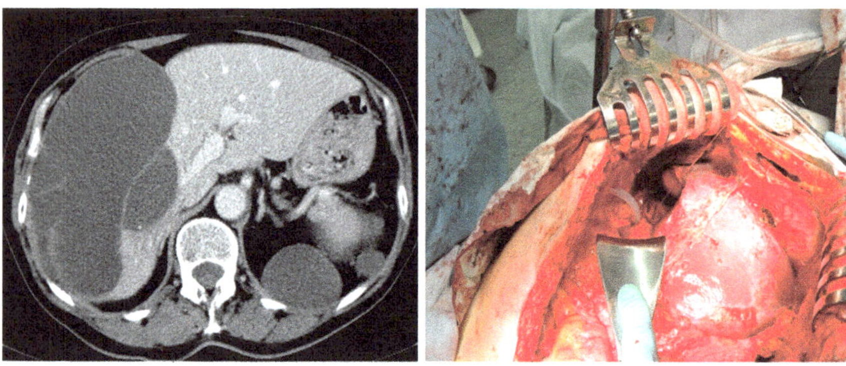

A B

Fig. 3.4 Removal of the tumor in the right upper hypochondrium. (**a**) CT sign; (**b**) Step of surgery

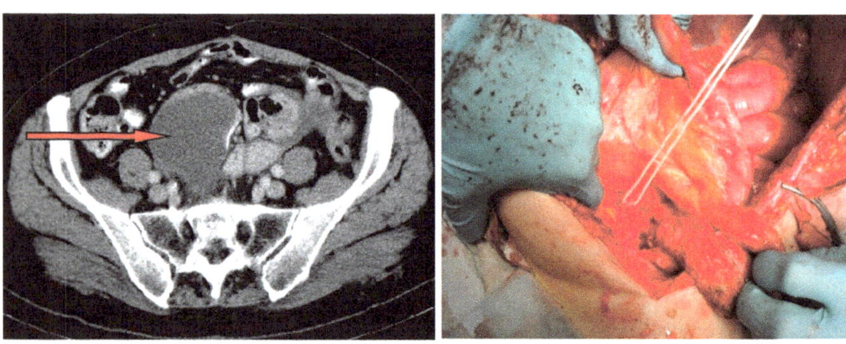

A B

Fig. 3.5 Preservation of the tumor capsule on the peritoneal small intestine in the pelvis due to the infiltration of the mesentery root, which led to the continued tumor growth in this area 6 months later. (**a**) CT sign; (**b**) Step of surgery

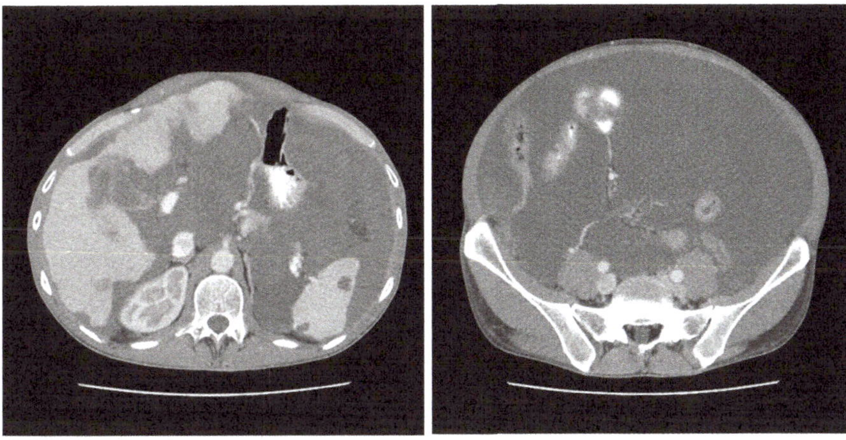

A B

Fig. 3.6 Peritoneal pseudomyxoma. (**a**) and (**b**) – CT signs

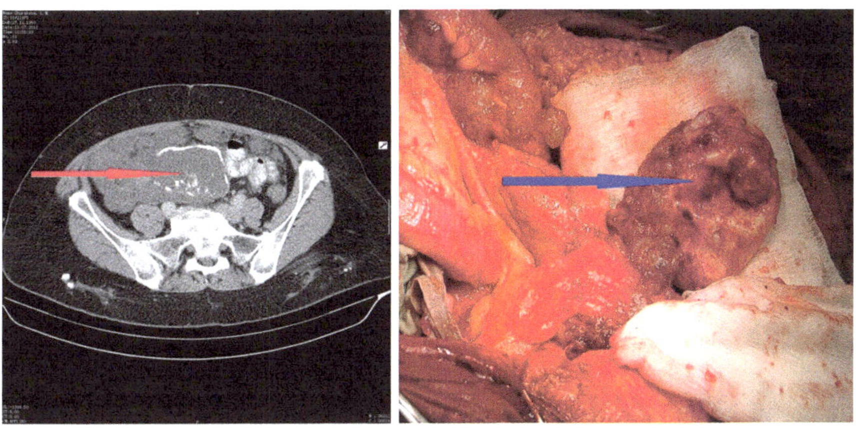

A B

Fig. 3.7 Tumor of the vermiform appendix, a calcified capsule. (**a**) CT sign; (**b**) Step of surgery

Another frequent CT sign of continued growth of pseudomyxoma after cytoreductive surgery is a localized accumulation of the fluid, which may have a mucinous or serous character due to the formation of tumor pseudocapsule (Fig. 3.8).

Evaluation of the completeness of cytoreduction after surgery was made according to two classifications:

1. «*Index of* ***Completeness of Cytoreduction***» (CC, Completeness of Cytoreduction) designed by Sugarbaker P.H [9].:

   CC-0 – maximum cytoreduction with removal of all "visible" disseminations.
   CC-1 – lesions of less than 2.5 mm in diameter after cytoreductive surgery.
   CC-2 – residual lesions ranging in size from 2.5 mm to 2.5 cm.
   CC-3 – remaining non-removed metastases of over 2.5 cm in diameter.

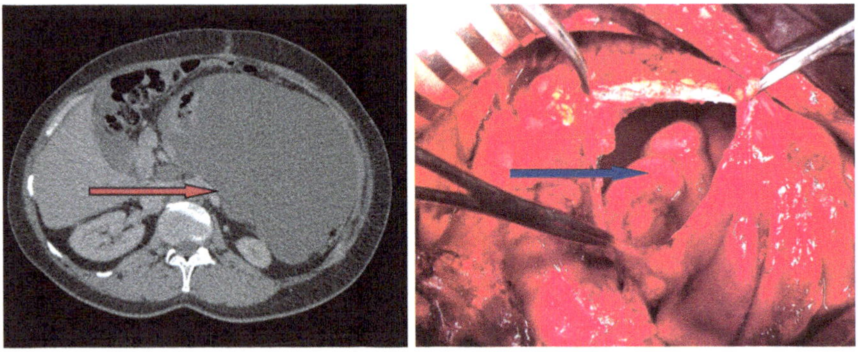

Fig. 3.8 Continued growth of pseudomyxoma, formation of pseudocapsule. (**a**) CT signs; (**b**) Step of surgery

2. Classification of the Japanese Gastric Cancer Association (1998), divides the completed intervention into three types:

Radical (type A) – no residual tumor with high probability of complete cure (R0).
Conditionally radical (type B) – no residual tumor (R0), but subclinical lesions are probable.
Palliative surgery (type C) – remaining microscopic (R1) or macroscopic (R2) residual tumor.

Despite the fact that this classification was designed for gastric tumors, we consider it more preferable due to its simplicity and less influence of subjective assessment.

3.2 Intraperitoneal Chemotherapy

There are two regimens of intraperitoneal chemotherapy:

1. Hyperthermic intraperitoneal chemotherapy (HIPEC) was performed in 31 patients with pseudomyxoma and 18 with mesothelioma.Until 2010 HIPEC was carried out with the device, designed at NN Blokhin Russian Cancer Research (Fig. 3.9).

All parts of this equipment for HIPEC were made on the base of modern medical devices of leading foreign and national manufacturers. Some elements required modification that was completed by the manufacturer of medical equipment at the appropriate plant. Such approach to the device construction was determined by the safety requirements for patients and staff when performing the procedure of hyperthermia. The entire system operates in semi-automatic mode, which allows maintaining accurate temperature and perfusion rate.

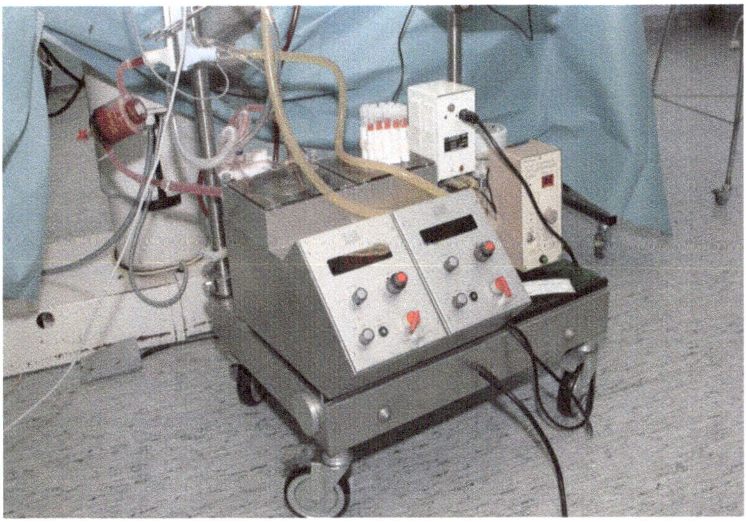

Fig. 3.9 HIPEC device

The principle of the HIPEC device operation implies the increase of the temperature of the perfusion fluid that circulates in a sterile circuit and flows through the abdominal drains for "inflow". This is achieved by passing through the heat exchanger of two circuits – "sterile" and "non-sterile". The latter is directly connected with the thermostat.

Perfusion fluid consisting of saline solution and chemotherapy drugs is prepared in the fluid collection unit, which is presented in the existing model as a 2-liter container where the level is controlled visually by the operator and is regulated by hand clamps. The perfused fluid is pumped (the pump design is based on the principle of peristaltic pumping of fluid through the tube) from the fluid collection unit through the filter into the thermostating unit where the fluid is heated up to 43–44 °C and flows into the patient's abdominal cavity. As the abdominal cavity is filled up, the overflow of the excess perfusate flows into the fluid collection unit with the following recirculation and heating. At a certain stage, the liquid current reaches a steady rate and the optimal regimen is 2–3 liters per minute, which at the optimal mode is 2–3 liters per minute. The process of perfusate temperature regimen is controlled by temperature sensors installed on the inlet and outlet drains. Information from these temperature sensors and temperature sensors from the patient is displayed on the medical screen, which allows the operator to establish the necessary temperature regimen. In this regard, HIPEC requires active operator's involvement, therefore the "human factor" plays an important role. HIC have performed with several Hyperthermic Intra-Peritoneal Chemotherapy Systems device is SunChip (France) (Fig. 3.10). It should be noted that HIC may be performed both in the "open" circuit, i.e., when the laparotomy wound is open and after its suturing – "closed" method. One of the variants of the "open" technique is the use of an expander that seals laparotomy access (Fig. 3.11). Polyethylene isolation is fixed on the skin of the anterior

Fig. 3.10 HIPEC is performed with a device SunChip

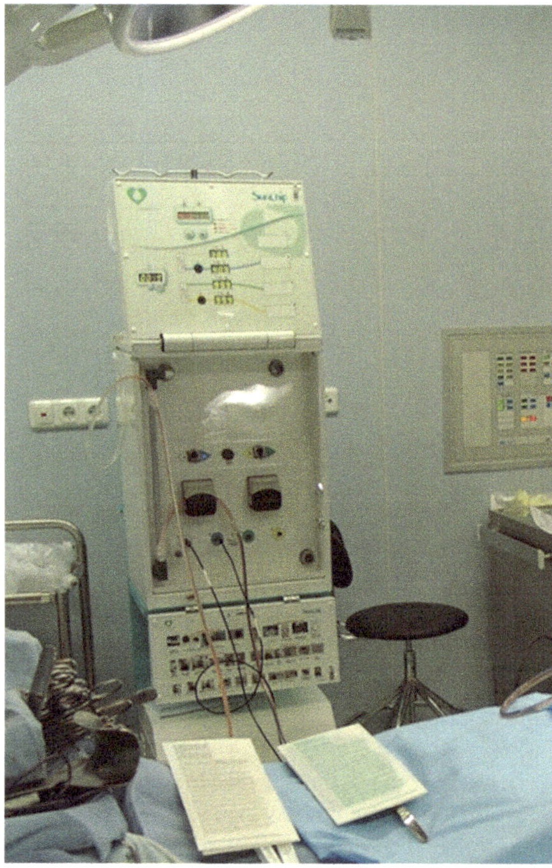

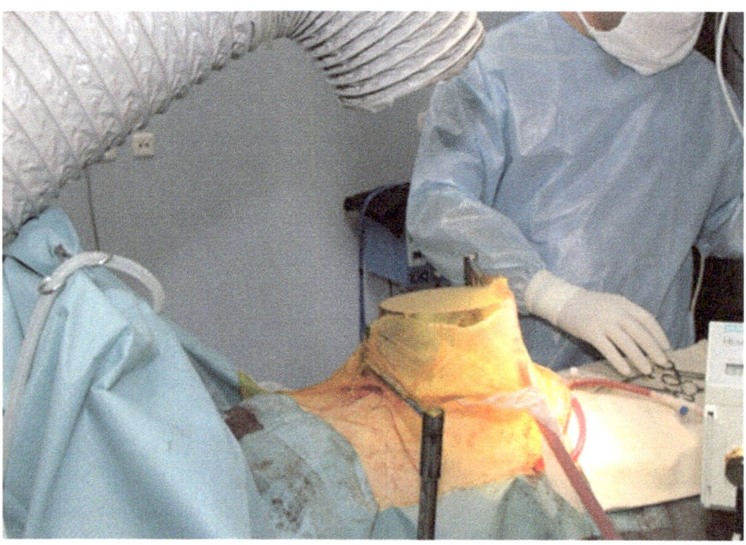

Fig. 3.11 "Open" method of HIPEC with expander

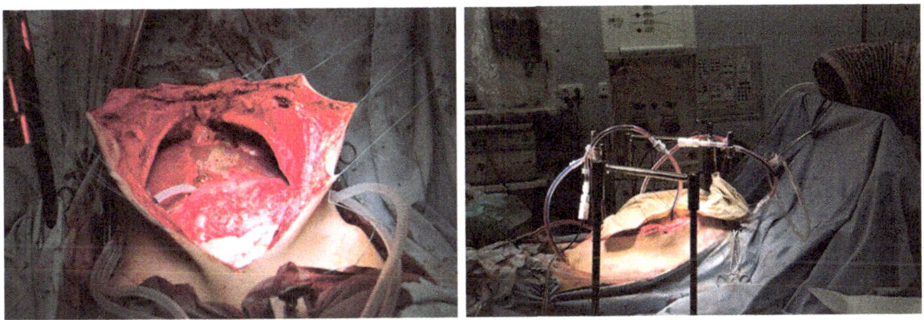

Fig. 3.12 "Open" method of HIPEC with Seigal retractor. (**a**) laparotomy; (**b**) installation of Sigal retractor

abdominal wall in order to prevent the evaporation of chemotherapeutic agents during the procedure. Another "open" method is to use Thompson or Segal retractors that fix the edges of the wound (Fig. 3.12).

The "closed" method involves the HIPEC procedure in a closed abdominal cavity through 4 drains 2 for inflow and 2 outflow of fluid (Fig. 3.13).

One variant of the «closed» method is a fully implantable system for intraperitoneal chemotherapy, consisting of a port and a catheter (Fig. 3.14).

HIPEC was performed immediately after surgery. Perfusion parameters (temperature, duration, cytostatics) were initially chosen empirically on the base of literature data and, later, on the base of our own analysis of survival of non-transformed and stem cells. Isotonic 0.9% NaCl solution was used in the amount of 5 liters intraperitoneally for perfusion, which made it possible to reduce the temperature gradient at the inflow and outflow by 1–1.5 °C, given a speed of 2–3 l/min.

Cisplatin in the dose of 100 mg/m^2 was used as a cytostatic. Prior to adding cytostatics into the perfusion medium, intravenous hydration was performed with 2 liters of iso-osmolar crystalloid (NaCl 0.9%), which determined a high rate of diuresis (>100 ml/h) in most cases. In case of decreased diuresis, furosemide was infused in multiple doses of 20 mg by intravenous infusion with blood electrolytes monitoring. Intravenous hyperhydration continued during the whole period of perfusion. The hydration amount was also controlled by central venous pressure. It is important to note that intraperitoneal infusion of cytostatics after extensive and traumatic surgery and then, defining the necessary water load are connected with certain difficulties due to altered preoperative parameters of BCV (circulating blood volume), hemoglobin level and blood electrolytes by the beginning of hyperthermic intraperitoneal chemotherapy. On the other hand, continuous intraoperative monitoring of central venous pressure, blood counts, urine output, ECG, blood pressure, and pulmonary ventilator reduces the risk of side effects.

The state of thermobalance during the procedure was studied by temperature sensors installed on the inlet and outlet ducts of the thermostat, as well as in the patient in multiple positions (oropharynx, rectum, skin). The average temperature of the perfusion solution was 43.6 ± 0.5 °C, the duration of the procedure – 60–90 min.

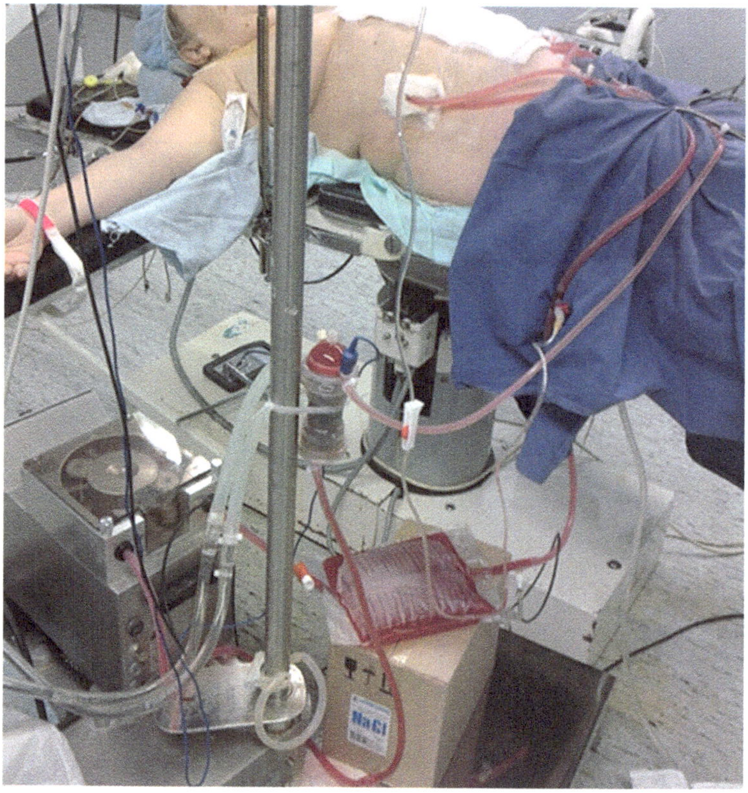

Fig. 3.13 "Closed" method of HIPEC

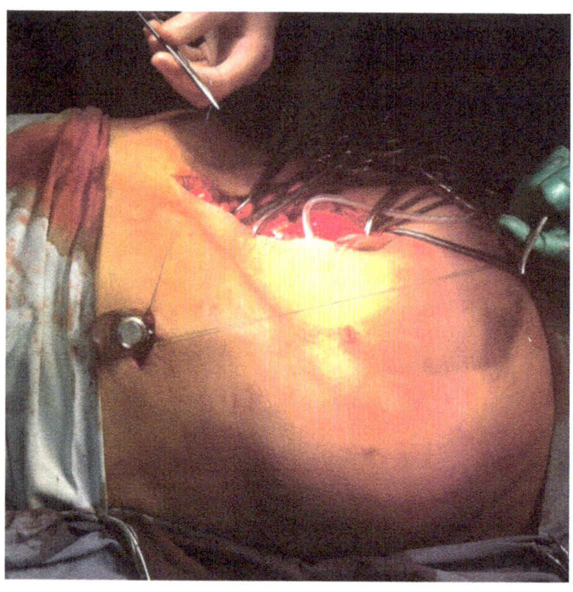

Fig. 3.14 "Closed" method of HIPEC

2. Chemotherapy with the laparoport, installed during the operation, was performed in patients with pseudomyxoma and with mesothelioma.

The indication for laparoport installation in patients with pseudomyxoma was suboptimal cytoreductive surgery provided that the patient had ascites. According to that, patients with pseudomyxoma had the laparoport installed in order to reduce ascites afterwards and improve quality of life.

Patients with mesothelioma also had ascites as an indication for laparoport installation, though in these cases it was used either after the optimum removal of the tumor, or after a diagnostic intervention.

3.3 Cytoreductive Surgery

The concept of "cytoreductive" surgery has existed for more than 20 years. Currently, it is widely used and reflects only one thing –maximum removal of the entire visible tumor.

The rationale for the potential effectiveness of such interventions can be:

1. cytoreductive surgery removes the main tumor bulk that has a low blood flow;
2. an opportunity of drug exposure to "small" tumors with high mitotic activity;
3. large tumors develop resistant types as a result of growing sites that were not affected by chemotherapy;
4. normalization of the patient's immune system after removal of the main tumor bulk, which the author explains by the decrease of immunosuppression induced by the tumor;
5. maximum removal of the tumor.

Initially, and currently, the term "cytoreductive surgery" is widely used in oncogynecology in the treatment of ovarian cancer [1].

In addition, there are concepts of primary, secondary and intermediate cytoreduction in oncogynecology. The latter is performed after a short course of induction chemotherapy.

To sum up, it should be mentioned that at present the term "cytoreductive surgery" is often used while analyzing the results of treatment of ovarian cancer [2–6, 7], colorectal cancer [8, 9], gastric cancer [10, 11], peritoneal pseudomyxoma and mesothelioma [12]. That is, in all forms of tumors with intraperitoneal dissemination. The authors agree that the interventions performed in carcinomatosis reduce the volume of the tumor and this improves survival rates.

Sugarbaker P. H [13]. has developed an operation subtotal peritonectomy in order to achieve maximum debulking and removal of all visually detected malignant lesions of the peritoneum. The procedure involves removal of 6 zones in the peritoneum:

- Peritonectomy of the upper-left quadrant of the abdominal cavity;
- Peritonectomy of the upper right quadrant of the abdominal cavity;

- Removal of the large omentum and spleen;
- Removal of the lesser omentum, peritoneum of the omentum sac and cholecystectomy;
- Removal of the pelvic peritoneum with possible removal of the sigmoid intestine with mesentery and uterus with appendages in women;
- Removal of the parietal peritoneum of the lateral canals and anterior abdominal wall.

Several classifications for assessment of cytoreduction completeness were suggested and the most popular is the "cytoreduction completeness index» (CC, Completeness of Cytoreduction), proposed by Sugarbaker P.H [13], which defines the following: CC-0 means maximum cytoreduction that removes all visual disseminated lesions, CC-1 implies lesions less than 2.5 mm in diameter found after cytoreductive surgery. CC-2 – remaining lesions of 2.5 mm – 2.5 cm, CC-3 means unremoved metastases of over 2.5 cm in diameter (Fig. 3.15).

We consider the above classification rather subjective and arbitrary. An alternative may be a classification designed by the Japanese Gastric Cancer Association (1998), which divides the effectiveness of the completed intervention in three types:

Radical (type A) – no residual tumor with high probability of complete cure (R0).
Conditionally-radical (type B) – no residual tumor (R0), but probably remaining subclinical lesions.
Palliative surgery (type C) – remaining microscopic (R1) or macroscopic (R2) residual tumors.

Although this classification was designed for gastric cancers, we consider it more advantageous due to its simplicity and less subjective opinion.

Moreover, it is important to notice that this type of operations especially require predominant removal of the parietal peritoneum since the main problem is often caused by carcinomatosis involving a significant part of the visceral peritoneum of the intestine and its mesentery, which essentially determines disease prognosis.

In this regard, we have designed and introduced an original technique of the cytoreductive surgery, which consists of several stages (Table 3.2).

I stage
Removal of greater omentum without preserving the arterial arcade at the greater curvature is due to the frequently developing continued tumor growth in the

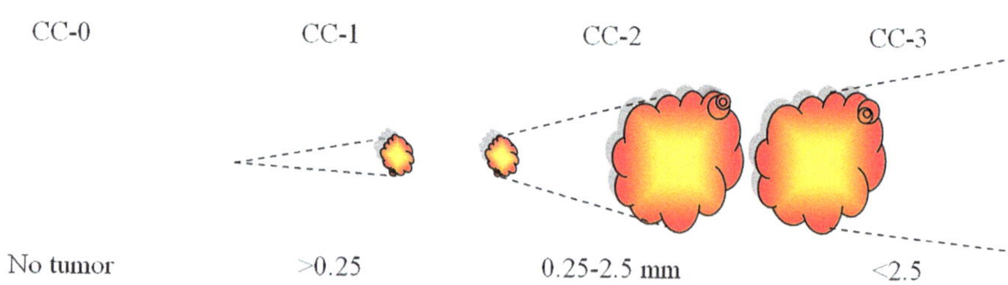

Fig. 3.15 Cytoreduction completeness index

Table 3.2 Stages of the cytoreductive surgery

I stage. Removal of greater and lesser omentums without preserving the arterial arcade
± splenectomy
± cholecystectomy
II stage. Removal of the tumor in mesogastric and hypogastric regions; extirpation of the uterus with appendages; appendectomy
±resection of the intestine
III stage. ± Removal of the peritoneum of the cupulas of diaphragm and lateral canals

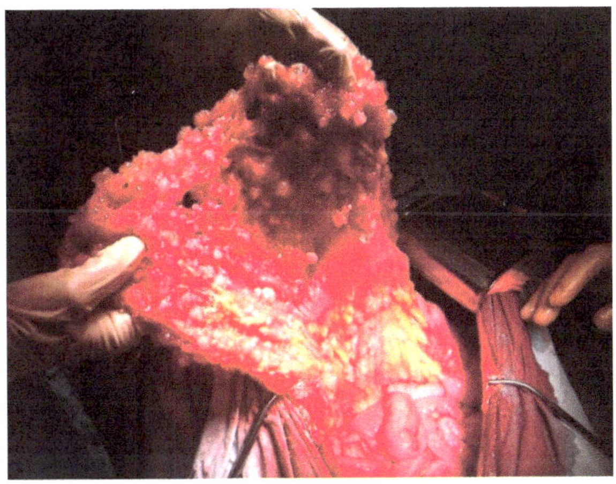

Fig. 3.16 Carcinomatosis of the greater omentum

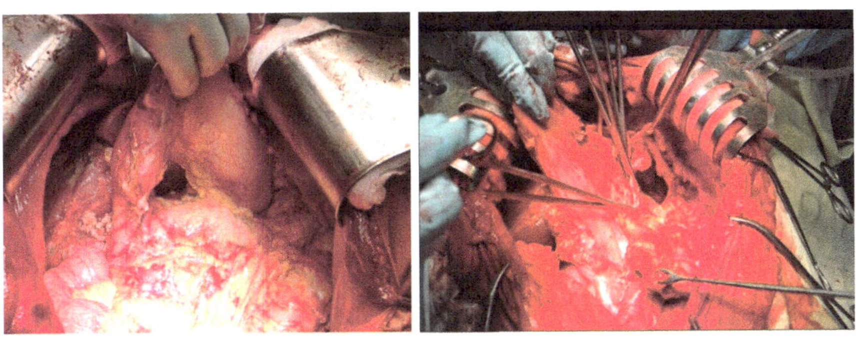

A *B*

Fig. 3.17 Removal of omentums: (**a**) the greater omentums; (**b**) lesser omentums

omentum stump. It is possible in case of malignancy to perform splenectomy and cholecystectomy at this stage.

We consider preventive cholecystectomy unreasonable. Not any patient of those who we analyzed had a pathologic affection of the gall bladder in the follow up, even in case of tumor infiltration in this region (Figs. 3.16 and 3.17).

II stage

Removal of the tumor lesions in mesogastric and hypogastric regions is performed with the mandatory extirpation of the uterus with appendages and appendectomy. Resection of the intestine of different volumes is possible at this stage if the patient has signs of partial mechanical obstruction, or if there is a threat of its development. Performing extirpation of the uterus with appendages in surgery of patients with pseudomyxoma and mesothelioma sometimes causes technical difficulties. The difficulties are connected with the frequent localization of tumor dissemination on the pelvic peritoneum, in the Douglas' cul-de-sac, and along the ligamentous apparatus of the uterus and appendages. It is recommended to start this stage with the mobilization of pelvic peritoneum and lateral canals and visualization of ureters and iliac vessels. This makes it safer to perform the subsequent stages of the operation (Figs. 3.18 and 3.19).

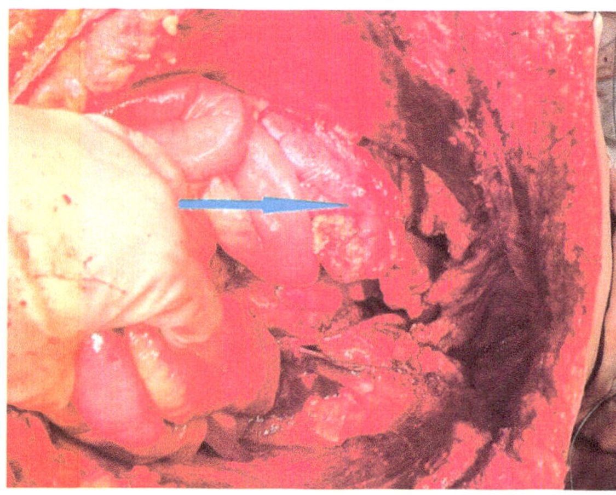

Fig. 3.18 Forming a descend-sigmoid anastomosis of the "side to side" type (arrow)

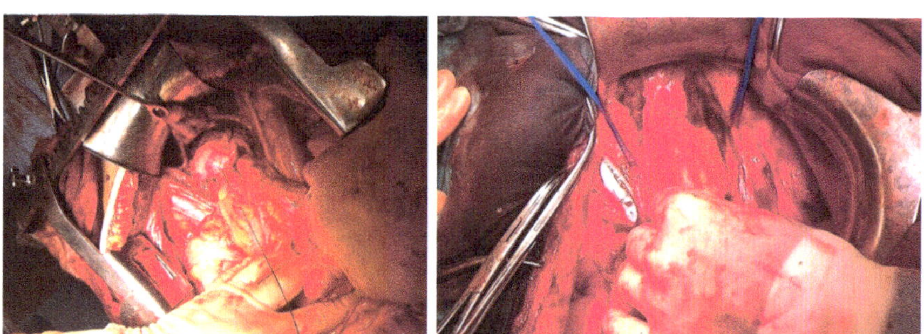

Fig. 3.19 Stages of the operation: (**a**) parietal pelvic peritonectomy; (**b**) visualization of the ureters

III stage
Removal of the peritoneum of the cupulas of diaphragm and lateral canals in case of carcinomatosis in these regions. This stage is not technically difficult (Fig. 3.20).

Given the wide wound surface, it is important to monitor hemostasis after surgery. The main idea of this approach is the maximum removal of tumor bulk and perfoming peritonectomy only of the affected areas of the peritoneum, and prevention of intestinal obstruction, due to compression as a consiquent of suboptimal cytoreduction. In addition, an important advantage of these interventions is the functional effect that influences the quality of life, i.e. formation of anastomoses in the abdominal cavity without persistent stoma.

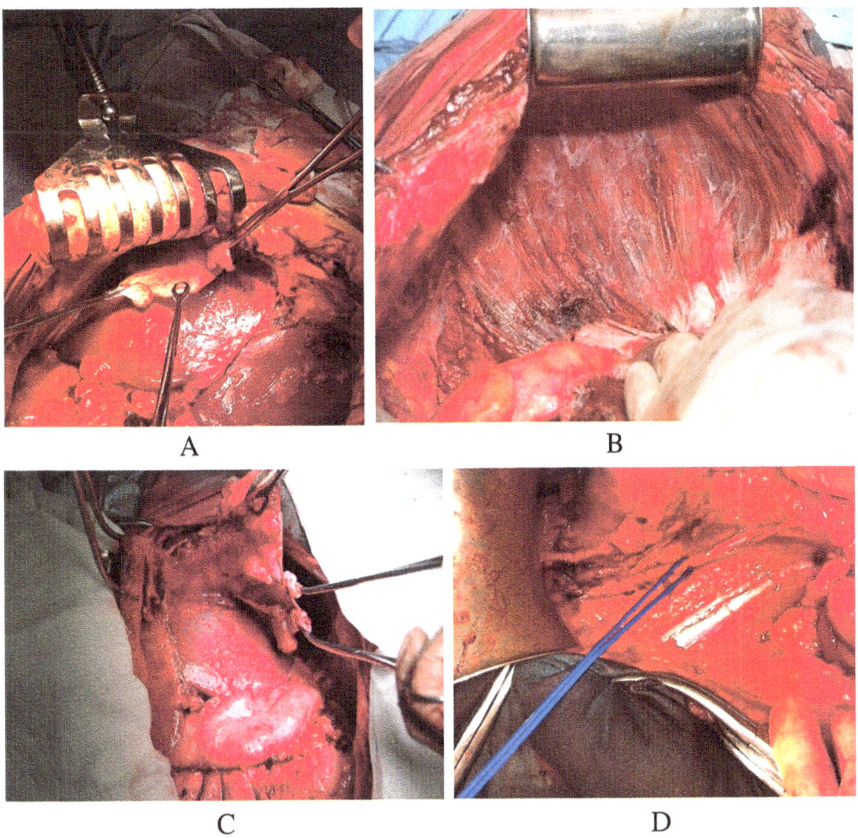

Fig. 3.20 Removal of the peritoneum of the cupulas of diaphragm and lateral canals in case of carcinomatosis in these regions: (**a**, **b**) peritonectomy of the right diaphragm cupula; (**c**) left diaphragm cupula; (**d**) left lateral canal

3.3.1 *Complications of Surgical Treatment*

Suppuration of postoperative wounds can develop in the early period. Daily sanation (debridement) of the wound, ointment bandages, and antibacterial therapy should be performed taking into account patient's sensitivity This treatment effectively results in healing by secondary intention. And the secondary seams are formed.

3.4 Intraperitoneal Chemotherapy

Patients with the identified intraperitoneal dissemination represent a very complex group in terms of developing strategy of treatment [14, 15]. Low survival rates, on the one hand, and a high risk of complications during the tumor progression on the other, make an alternative – either to perform cytoreductive surgery or to conduct systemic chemotherapy. These methods can also complement each other. Cytoreductive palliative surgery may be motivated by a possibility to prevent fatal complications (bleeding, perforation, obstruction) and to reduce the tumor bulk in order to improve chemotherapy effectiveness. On the other hand, Yonemura Y. (2001), reports that systemic chemotherapy in patients with peritoneal malignant dissemination is limited by poor ability of cytostatics to penetrate in the peritoneum due to peritoneal plasmatic barrier that includes a complex of barriers for diffusion of different agents and involves endothelium, mesothelium and interstitial tissues.

Low efficiency of therapy of patients with pseudomixoma and mesothelioma determine the need for up-to-date methods of combined treatment that reduce the risk of early intraperitoneal relapse.

A key point for significant treatment improvement in intraperitoneal administration of cytostatics is the prolonged exposure to the drug in the abdominal cavity, which ensures its high concentration. The experiments with mitomycin C demonstrated that substances with high molecular weight were kept in the abdominal cavity for a long period [12]. The author makes a conclusion that the contact of peritoneum and a cytostatic may be extended by intraperitoneal but not intravenous administration. Pharmacokinetic studies have shown that the half-life of different chemotherapy drugs eliminated from the abdominal cavity varies for etoposide, cisplatin and mitomycin with 4.2 ± 1.8; 0.85 ± 0.26 and 1.0 hours, respectively [16, 17]. Another study showed that concentrations of 5-fluorouracil, mitomycin C, doxorubicin and cisplatin in the abdominal cavity after intraperitoneal administration exceed their concentrations in blood plasma in 250, 75, 500 and 20 times, respectively [18, 19].

Weisberger described the first intraperitoneal administration of chemotherapy in 1955 [20]. To date, a large experience of various intraperitoneal chemotherapy regimens has been collected in a lot of international studies. Special formulations of chemotherapeutic drugs of prolonged action were designed to achieve a more continuous and uniform infusion of cytotoxics into the peritoneal cavity [21–24]. Kurita A [25], Ohta K [26] et al. report the design of special tanks through which the drug is released into the abdominal cavity for a long time. In addition, intraperitoneal chemotherapy differs in time and in relation to the stage of the operation: induction intraperitoneal chemotherapy (IPC) in patients with peritoneal dissemination [26], intraoperative chemotherapy, when cytostatics are administered at the end of the operation [13], early postoperative intraperitoneal chemotherapy [27, 28], and a combination of intraperitoneal and systemic postoperative chemotherapy [29].

According to the recent years' literature reports intraperitoneal chemotherapy with hyperthermia (HIC) is one of the promising methods of combined treatment of pseudomixoma and peritoneal mesothelioma.

Sugarbaker P.H [13] presents a number of advantages of hyperthermia in the manual of cytoreductive surgery and intraperitoneal chemotherapy. According to the author, hyperthermia has not only its own cytotoxicity against the tumor as compared to normal tissues, but also increases the penetration of chemotherapeutic drugs in the tissue and therefore enhances the effect of chemotherapy. The latter is explained by the fact that hyperthermia activates the process of peroxidation of tumor cell membranes with an increase of their permeability [30]. In addition, tumor cells experience a delay of redox processes as a result of a pH decrease and an increase in lysosomal function [31]. J. R. Oleson et al. [32] report the data on the greater cytotoxic effect of hyperthermia on tumor cells than normal cells.

Issels R. D. (2008) also presented the data on the possible efficacy of hyperthermia in his preclinical analysis. The author emphasizes the improved effectiveness of higher temperatures, which in combination with chemotherapy has a pronounced cytotoxic effect and, in addition, is able to strengthen the immune response [33].

Thus, the analysis of the literature data shows that both treatment components are synergistic, potentiating their cytotoxic effect on tumor cells, as well as the depth of drug penetration into the tissues.

The first combination of hyperthermia and chemotherapy was performed by Spratt et al. [34] in a young patient with pseudomyxoma peritonei. Chemoperfusion included thiophosphamide dissolved in 1.5 L of Ringer solution infused for 1 hour at the temperature of 42 °C. No complications were registered. The patient lived over 3 years with good quality of life.

3.4.1 *Parameters of HIPEC*

The choice of perfusion solution, the chemotherapeutic agent, plays an important role in the clearance of the drug from the abdominal cavity. However, the chemical composition of the solution is not the only factor affecting the pharmacokinetics and penetration of chemotherapy drugs into the tumor. Other factors, such as the concentration of cytostatics in the perfusion solution and its volume should be taken into account as well [35, 36].

Main characteristics of different types of perfusion solutions

1. Isotonic sodium chloride solution and dextrose solution. Torres IJ [37] considers that it is impossible to maintain high intraperitoneal volume of the liquid for a long time when using this solution and it is rapidly absorbed due to the low molecular weight.

2. Hypotonic solutions. The experimental data demonstrated that it is possible to increase the accumulation of cisplatin in tumor cells and increase the immediate cytotoxicity when using hypotonic solution [38–40]. On the other hand, intraoperative infusion of heated oxaliplatin solution in the hypotonic solution resulted in an increased frequency of unexplained postoperative peritoneal bleeding and showed no advantages in pharmacokinetics [41].
3. Hypertonic solutions enable a longer maintenance of a large volume of intraperitoneal liquid [42]. The main disadvantage is a decrease in the drug concentration [43].
4. Isotonic solutions with high molecular weight. McArdle C.S [44]. reports the data demonstrating that these solutions facilitate maintaining a large intraperitoneal volume for a long time and reduce drug clearance from the abdominal cavity. However, the decrease in drug clearance from the abdominal cavity does not imply an increase of the contact the cytostatic and the tumor.

Temperature of the perfusion solution.

The literature reports various temperature regimens, namely: from 40 °C to 41°C [45], from 41 to 43°C [46], from 41 to 42.5°C [47], 42°C [48], from 42 to 43°C [49] and from 42 to 45°C [50].

In order to determine the optimal temperature level during perfusion it is necessary to discuss the factors of interaction between high temperature and chemotherapy and, in addition, the risk of unfavorable effects. The synergistic effect between cytostatic and temperature starts at 39 °C and increases with rising temperature. The study of cell culture at 45 °C showed that cytotoxicity of chemotherapeutic agents is much higher than that at the temperatures of 41° or 42 °C. Thus, it is theoretically advisable to apply high temperatures, limited only by clinical tolerance [51]. In addition, the literature provides the data of the successful infusion with "heavy" temperature regimen in the range of 45–47 °C of the perfusion solution for 90 min resulting in a rather satisfying tolerance [52]. At the same time, according to the author, the temperature in the tissues varies significantly from 41.7 °C in the liver to 42.8 °C in the stomach and is associated with the speed of blood circulation in the organ. We have found only one paper of the study of thermal resistance, which was performed on animals (rats). It established that the optimal temperature regime was 44 °C for 30 minutes [47].

However, the analysis of literature data still does not give completely clear requirements for the most appropriate solution temperature, duration of hyperthermia, the drugs to be used and their concentrations.

3.4.2 Chemotherapy Drugs for Intraperitoneal Infusion

In 2006 the National Institute for Cancer Research in Milan held a conference on peritoneal carcinomatosis [51]. Among other things, the speakers discussed issues related to chemotherapy drugs for intraperitoneal infusion. The experts included cytostatics (or a combination of drugs) as a phase of scientific research. According to most experts, only cisplatin and mitomycin C can be used in clinical practice for intraperitoneal infusion.

According to the joined experts' opinions the presented cytostatics can be divided into several groups:

1. Drugs that are inappropriate for HIPEC – paclitaxel and 5-fluorouracil [53].
2. Drugs that refer to the stage of an experimental study – gemcitabine, mitoxantrone, etoposide, docetaxel, cisplatin+interferon alpha, carboplatin+interferon alpha.
3. Drugs of the phase I study: melphalan, irinotecan, carboplatin, oxaliplatin+irinotecan.
4. Drugs of the phase III study: oxaliplatin, combination of oxaliplatin (i.p.) + leucovorin (i.v.) + 5-fluorouracil (i.v.).
5. Drugs that are available for clinical practice: doxorubicin, cisplatin, mitomycin C, 5-FU, cisplatin with doxorubicin, cisplatin with mitomycin C.

However, the presented above classification is very conditional, since currently there is no consensus on which of the cytostatics, or their combination, should be used for intraperitoneal chemotherapy. In addition, to date, rational doses of intraperitoneal chemotherapy drugs have not been determined yet.

3.5 Combined Treatment of Patients with Pseudomixoma Peritonei

Conventional treatment of patients with pseudomyxoma involved multiple repeated surgical interventions aimed at relieving the disease symptoms. There are observations which report asymptomatic course of the disease for many years, although the disease is almost always progressing, often with the development of symptoms of the intestinal obstruction.

In 1994 Cough reported 31% of 10-year survival in the group of 56 patients with pseudomyxoma peritonei, who underwent periodic interventions to reduce tumor bulk and selective intraperitoneal radiation therapy or chemotherapy. In 2005 T. J. Miner et al. [54, 55] presented the data of 21% of 10-year survival in the group of 97 patients with pseudomyxoma peritonei, who also underwent periodic surgical interventions to reduce the tumor bulk in combination with systemic chemotherapy and/or with an intermitting intraperitoneal infusion of 5 –fluorouracil.

Later, a lot of papers were published describing the studies of the effectiveness of the combination of cytoreductive surgery with intraperitoneal chemotherapy and hyperthermia [55, 56]. One of them analyzes 174 observations of patients with pseudomixoma, who received combined treatment after non-radical operations. The total 5-year survival rate reached 15%. On the other hand, optimal cytoreductive surgery which removes all visible lesions can enhance the overall 5-year survival rate up to 84% [57].

In 2012 a paper was published that summarized the experience of pseudomixoma treatment in 16 medical centers in Europe. The study included 2298 patients. The overall 5-year survival with optimal tumor removal was more than 80%. It should be noted that most surgeries (more than 80%) resulted in an optimal tumor debulking, which, according to the authors who analyzed this work, indicated a careful selection of patients for combined treatment, and/or a high level of surgery [55].

In 2010 Glehen O, et al. [58] reported a large retrospective study of the efficacy of non-ovarian carcinomatosis treatment that involved perioperative chemotherapy (intraoperative hyperthermal chemotherapy and early postoperative intraperitoneal chemotherapy) and cytoreductive surgery. The analysis included 1290 patients of 25 centers. The HIPEC procedure was performed in 1154 cases. The number of patients with pseudomyxoma accounted for 301 people. The total 3-and 5-year survival rate was 85 and 73%, respectively. The median was not achieved. Although the authors made a detailed analysis of preoperative data (PCI, Gilly, histological type, etc.), the long-term results were given for the total group of patients, which we consider is not quite appropriate. The authors reported that the proportion of optimal cytoreductive surgeries (CC0) was more than 70% and 17% were classified as CC1 (tumor less than 2.5 mm), while advanced carcinomatosis (type 3 and 4 Gilly) was determined in more than 50% of patients. Besides that, there was no accurate description of the cases which were treated with hyperthermal intraperitoneal intraoperative chemotherapy, and which underwent early postoperative chemotherapy, which therapy scheme was used (the authors mention three of them), and whether "open" or "closed" HIPEC technique was performed. The average perfusion time was 59.5 ± 28.7 min, the perfusion temperature was 42.5% ± 0.8 °C, which is currently the standard parameters. In general, overall survival rates were quite sufficient that demonstrates the effectiveness of combined pseudomixoma treatment by cytoreductive surgery and intraperitoneal chemotherapy. The summary of the literature analyses of the treatment results of patients with pseudomyxoma are presented in Table 3.3.

Table 3.3 Treatment results of patients with pseudomixoma

Author	Number of Patients	Therapy	Survival
Glehen M. and Sugabaker P. [57]	N = 174	76 EPIC+CRS 61 IPCH+CRS	Median – 20.5 months. 3-year – 34% 5-year – 15%
Gough et al. (Mayo Cinic) [59]	N = 56	CRS CCR0 33%	5-year – 53% Recurrence – 97%
Miner et al. (Memorial SK) [55]	N = 97	67 CRS 30 CRS+ IPCH CCR0 53%	10- year – 21% Recurrence – 88%
D. Elias [58]	N = 301	255 CRS + HIPEC CCR0 73%	5- year – 75% 10- year – 55%
Chua et al. [56]	N = 2298	668 CRS + HIPEC+ EPIC 1382 CRS + HIPEC 44 CRS+ EPIC 203 CRS CCR0–1˃80%	10- year – 63% 15- year – 59%

Notice: *CCR* completeness of cytoreduction, *EPIC* early postoperative intraperitoneal chemotherapy, *HIPEC* hyperthermic intraperitoneal chemotherapy, *IPCH* intraperitoneal chemotherapy, *CRS* cytoreduction surgeon, *PIC* perioperative intraperitoneal chemotherapy

On the whole, the analysis of the presented studies demonstrated the best survival rates of the combined approach: cytoreductive surgery in combination with intraperitoneal chemotherapy provided optimal tumor removal was achieved. The latter is confirmed by M. Glehen's study [60], where, despite the intraperitoneal chemotherapy, the results of non-radical interventions were worse than after CCR0 operations with no chemotherapy.

Recently, an interesting paper has been published that presents a comparative analysis of pseudomixoma treatment by intraperitoneal chemotherapy with hyperthermia versus surgical treatment alone. Wheeler et al. [61] demonstrats that the treatment results with disseminated peritoneal adenomucinosis are similar in both groups of patients.

3.6 Combined Treatment of Patients with Peritoneal Mesothelioma

The standard treatment option for patients with peritoneal mesothelioma, including palliative and symptomatic operations and systemic chemotherapy, demonstrates disappointing results with a median survival of 6–15 months [62–67].

Low treatment effectiveness also results from treatment of patients with mesothelioma by only systemic chemotherapy, which is usually performed with platinum drugs in combination with other cytostatics, and according to some authors, the median survival is less than 15 months, and 5-year survival does not reach 30% [68].

Standard schemes of systemic chemotherapy for mesothelioma treatment:

- Pemetrexed+cisplatin
- Gemcitabine+oxaliplatin
- Raltitrexed+oxaliplatin
- Navelbine+cisplatin

Moreover, intra-abdominal chemotherapy alone, with no surgical stage, did not show any significant improvement in survival while the median of 5–9 months [69, 70]. Mansini et al. [71] analyzed the treatment results of 81 patients with mesothelioma: 30 patients underwent surgery and 40 received systemic chemotherapy. Median survival of these patients reached 13 months only.

Over the last 20 years cytoreductive surgery of P. Sugarbaker's technique in combination with hyperthermic intraperitoneal chemotherapy has become a popular approach to treatment of intraperitoneally disseminated ovarian cancer, pseudomyxoma, and colorectal cancer. This approach has become also relevant for peritoneal mesothelioma treatment, mainly due to the intraperitoneal tumor dissemination.

Blackham A.U. et al. [72] reported the results of peritoneal mesothelioma treatment of 38 patients with HIPEC. The average age of patients was 55 years, the optimal cytoreduction was achieved in 22 patients (R0/1 or R2a, residual tumor ≤5 mm), median survival was 40.8 months, and 3 – and 5-year survival reached 56% and 17%, respectively. Interestingly, the comparative analysis of mitomycin C

Table 3.4 Results of treatment of peritoneal mesothelioma in combination with HIPEC Patient number Median of overall survival

Study	Number of Patients	Median of overall survival	Survival	
			3-year	5-year
Blackham [73]	38	41	56%	17%
Brigand [90]	15	36	43%	29%
Baratti [75]	83	44	–	50%
Feldman [95]	49	92	59%	59%
Yan [87]	100	52	55%	46%
Kluger [76]	47	55	62%	49%
Yan [74]	401	53	60%	47%
Tudor [77]	20	30	46%	–
Helm [80]	1047	–	59%	42%
Robella [78]	42	65	–	44%
Magge [79]	65	46,2	–	39%

and cisplatin efficiency showed the advantage of the latter – the 3-year survival rate after cisplatin therapy accounted for 80% versus 42% after mitomycin C therapy.

Another large multicenter study presented the results of treatment of 405 patients [73]. 318 patients (79%) had epithelioid histological type of tumor. Metastases in lymph nodes were detected in 25 (6%) patients. The average peritoneal carcinomatosis index (PCI) was 20. Optimal cytoreductive surgery was achieved in 187 patients (46%), and HIPEC was performed in 92% of cases. Median overall survival reached 53 months, 3 – and 5-year survival rates were 60% and 47%, respectively.

In 2015 Helm JH et al. [74] reported a meta-analysis of more than 20 scientific publications on mesothelioma, including 1047 patients. The average age of patients was 51, with 59% of females, and mean PCI = 19 (16 to 23). Optimal cytoreduction (CC0–1) was achieved in 67% of cases. 1 -, 3- and 5-year survival rates were 84, 59, and 42%, respectively. The authors observed the improvement of survival rates after intraperitoneal chemotherapy.

Summary of the literature data on the mesothelioma treatment are presented in Table 3.4.

On the whole, the literature analysis of the treatment of pseudomixoma peritonei and peritoneal mesothelioma has demonstrated the advantage of combined treatment of these tumors, which includes optimal cytoreductive surgery and one of the regimens of intraperitoneal chemotherapy.

3.7 Prognostic Factors for Peritoneal Pseudomyxoma and Mesothelioma

Combined treatment of peritoneal carcinomatosis for the last 20 years resulted in defining factors that have their impact on disease prognosis. We consider it important to analyze prognostic factors before planning your own similar study, since that will highlight the main factors which cannot be neglected when designing a therapy strategy.

The literature review suggests that similar factors affect the prognosis of peritoneal pseudomyxoma and mesothelioma, therefore, we do not separate them in connection with the nosology. A single-factor analysis of a multicenter study involving 1290 patients (Glehen O, 59) [58] could not identify the factors that increase the risk of complications. Such parameters as the type of a cytostatic agent, its concentration, temperature and duration of perfusion were not taken into account due to significant differences in various medical centers. However, the multi-factor analysis revealed 3 major factors affecting the immediate results of treatment: the patient's age, PCI index and the medical center where the treatment was performed [80–82].

An additional factor affecting the frequency of complications is the patient's age (over 70 years) and the grade of tumor dissemination, evaluated by the PCI classification. It has been noticed that in case of a larger lesion of the peritoneum, the surgeon has to perform a more extended surgery, which increases the risk of complications. On the other hand, it is necessary to take into account the side effects of cytostatics (neutropenia, anemia, renal failure, vomiting, etc.), which alone can increase the risk of developing a surgical complication. Although in practice it is not always clear what exactly caused the complication (toxicity of chemotherapy or surgery).

The multivariate analysis of another multicenter study (Tristan D. Yan) of peritoneal mesothelioma identified 4 main prognostic factors, such as epithelial tumor type (P = .001), absence of metastases in lymph nodes (P = .001), the completeness of cytoreduction (P = .001), and HIC (P = .002) [73]. In fact, epithelioid histological type of mesothelioma is associated with a better prognosis than sarcomatoid and biphase variants [83–85]. Metastasis into the lymph nodes is not typical for mesothelioma or pseudomixoma, but is also a reliable factor of the negative prognosis [86]. Yan et al. [86] reported seven cases of metastases of mesothelioma into lymph nodes. Median survival rate of these patients was 6 months, 1- and 2-year survival rate was 43% and 0%, respectively. 93 patients had no metastases in lymph nodes; median survival was 59 months, 5- and 7-year survival rates were 50% and 43%. The authors made a conclusion about the importance of intraoperative evaluation of retroperitoneal lymph nodes status.

Another very important factor of the prognosis should be considered the completeness of cytoreduction and in this terms, a "residual tumor". It is established that the optimal cytoreduction is CCR0–1, where the remaining lesions are not more than 2.5 mm. Such situation is obviously explained by the following: firstly, the risk of complications decreases as a result of the reduced tumor bulk, and due to the possible torpid course of the disease it independently provides an increase in the survival rate; secondly, it is proved that the smaller the thickness of the tumor, the more effective the impact of cytostatics of intraperitoneal infusion, while theoretically hyperthermia increases the depth of chemotherapy penetration by reducing the tumor density [83, 84, 86–90].

Elias (2010) performed a detailed analysis of prognostic factors for pseudomixoma peritonei. The study included analysis of the case histories of 301 patients. The author reported that the multi-factor analysis revealed the main prognostic factors, such as the degree of intraperitoneal dissemination (p = 0.004), the degree of malignancy (p = 0.03), gender (p = 0.02), and HIPEC (p = 0.04). However, a single-factor analysis of 206 patients after optimal cytoreduction, the only prognosis factor was the grade of intraperitoneal dissemination (p = 0.004) [57]. Yan et al. also reported about a possible impact of the patient's gender in their study, with the better prognosis for women. This may be explained by the suggestion that when women refer to a gynecologist, the disease can be detected at an earlier stage during gynecological examination [83]. On the other hand, the studies showed that women had more favorable histological types of peritoneal mesothelioma [91], however, the author mentioned that the patient's gender determined the disease prognosis only in case of a single factor analysis and this relation was not confirmed in a multi-factor analysis.

In general, literature analysis showed that the main prognostic factors for pseudomyxoma and mesothelioma are histological tumor type, the grade of intraperitoneal dissemination (PCI), completeness of cytoreduction (CCR), and intraperitoneal chemotherapy.

3.8 Complications of Combined Treatment – Cytoreductive Surgery, Intraperitoneal Chemotherapy

Cytoreductive surgery combined with intraperitoneal chemotherapy is associated with a high risk of complications in the postoperative period for several reasons, such as:

- firstly, in case of advanced carcinomatosis, the surgeon is forced to manipulate almost in all parts of the abdominal cavity, which causes extensive surgical trauma for the patient. The scope of surgical intervention often includes resection of the stomach or intestine, extirpation of uterus with appendages, extended removal of the parietal peritoneum in the area of the diaphragm domes, lateral channels and in the pelvis.
- secondly, the independent cytotoxic effect of chemotherapy drugs is important, the side effects of which can be enhanced by hyperthermia and the surgical trauma [51, 92–94].

On the other hand, combination of cytoreductive surgery with loco-regional chemotherapy makes it difficult to identify the true cause of the complication. For example, anemia in the postoperative period may be associated with bleeding or with the side effects of chemotherapy (inhibition of hematopoiesis), or simultaneous influence of these factors. Kusamura S. et al. [95] found that cisplatin at the dose of over 240 mg used in HIC, was an independent risk factor for increasing frequency of surgical complications of combined treatment (cytoreductive surgery + HIPEC). Contrary to this, most authors suggest classification of complications associated with surgery in a different way from complications caused by chemotherapy.

Table 3.5 Classification of surgical complications

Grade	Definition
Grade I	Any deviation from the normal course of the postoperative period with no need of pharmacological, surgical, endoscopic and radiological interventions.
	Acceptable therapeutic regimens are as following – antiemetic drugs, antipyretics, analgesics, diuretics, electrolytes and physiotherapy. This grade also includes a wound infection, cut "at the bedside".
Grade II	Treatment requires the drugs in addition to those listed for complications of grade I. It also includes blood transfusions and total parenteral nutrition.
Grade III	Surgical, endoscopic or radiological interventions are needed.
IIIa	Interventions with no general anesthesia
IIIb	Interventions under general anesthesia.
Grade IV	Life-threatening complications (including central nervous system complications) requiring extensive care in the intensive care unit.
IVa	Dysfunction of one organ (including the need for dialysis).
IVb	Multi organ failure.
Grade V	Patient's death.

Currently, most authors use the classification proposed by ClavienPA with co-authors to evaluate complications, which consists of five grades – from minor complications that do not require complex therapeutic measures (grade I) to hospital mortality (grade V) [96] (Table 3.5).

Other authors report the use of a relatively simple classification proposed by Bozzetti F [95, 97, 98]. This classification includes 4 grades:

Grade 1 – no complications
Grade 2 – «small» complications: wound infection, urinary tract infection, pancreatitis, intestinal obstruction, deep vein thrombosis.
Grade 3 – «large» complications: required repeated surgery or extensive care.
Grade 4 – hospital mortality.

Kusamura S. et al. [95] reported the frequency of complications in case of using this classification. The analysis involved 209 patients with different grades of carcinomatosis. The results revealed that over a 30 days' period mortality was 0.9%, complications of grade 3–4 accounted for 12%. However, the presented classifications cannot estimate the degree of chemotherapy toxicity in HIPEC. At present most authors use the WHO classification. Yoo CH [99] reported that hematologic toxicity after several courses of intraperitoneal chemotherapy, including mitomycin C, cisplatin, and 5–fluorouracil of grade 3–4 manifested anemia in 6.6% of patients, leukopenia – 13.2%, thrombocytopenia – 15.3%. Another study showed the second or higher grade of haematological toxicity was 8.2% [29].

The analysis of the immediate results of cytoreductive operations in combination with intraperitoneal chemotherapy in specialized centers showed that the frequency

Table 3.6 Frequency of complications in cytoreductive surgery + HIPEC

Author	Complications of III-IV degree	Frequency of repeated surgery	Stpsis	Intestinal fistula	Abscess	The failure of the anastomosis
Elias et al. [58]	52%	23%	–	23%	8%	0%
Van Leenwen et al. [102]	43%	18%	8%	5%	9%	4%
Rufian et al. [103]	36%	6%	0%	0%	0%	0%
Gusani et al. [104]	30%	–	4%	2%	4%	7%
Clemente et al. [105]	23%	0%	0%	0%	7.7%	0%
Robella et al. [78]	35.7%	–	–	–	–	–
Magge et al. [79]	35%	–	–	–	–	–

Table 3.7 Causes of fatal outcomes after cytoreductive surgery + HIPEC

Author	The average bed-day in hospital	Average bed-day in ICU	Mortality %	Causes of death
Glehen et al. [57]	11.8	–	3.2	Septic shock; pulmonary embolism, peritonitis, multiple organ failure, aplastic anemia, acute renal failure
Elias et al.[58]	24	–	4	Aspiration pneumonia, mesenteric thrombosis
Van Leenwen et al. [102]	15	1	1	Insult
Sugabaker et al. [14]	21	–	2	The failure of the anastomosis, pulmonary embolism, neutropenia

of complications varied from 12% to 52%, mortality – 0 to 17% (Tables 3.6, 3.7). The reasons that increased the risk of complications included the following: the grade of intraperitoneal dissemination, duration of the operation, the history of previous surgical interventions, the number of formed anastomoses and doses of chemotherapy drugs [93, 94, 100, 101].

Glehen and co-authors [60] analyzed the frequency of complications of combined treatment in the multicenter study that involved 1290 patients and showed that postoperative mortality was 4.1% (n = 52), and the causes of death were: multiple organ failure (n = 11), septic shock (n = 10), pulmonary complications (n = 10), intestinal fistula or peritonitis (n = 4), pulmonary embolism (n = 2), cardiac pathology (n = 5), hemorrhagic shock (n = 2), haematological toxicity (n = 2) and acute renal failure (n = 2). The frequency of complications of grades III-IV was 33.6% (n = 403). 173 (14%) patients required repeated surgery. The most frequent surgical complication was intestinal fistula (9.7%, n = 123), complication of chemotherapy – neutropenia (13.3%, n = 178). The average in hospital period was 24.1 ± 17.4 days. A single-factor analysis identified the following causes that may affect the frequency of complications: gender, carcinomatosis cause (etiology), the second or third surgery in a row, the previous neoadjuvant chemotherapy, synchronous liver resection during surgery and the duration of the operation. The impact of intraperitoneal chemotherapy parameters such as the cytostatic type, dose, perfusate temperature could not be taken into account due to the fact that different regimes were used in different centers. A multi-factor regression analysis included the following factors significantly increasing the risk of complications and mortality: age (frequency of complications increased with age), the grade of intraperitoneal dissemination (PCI) and the center where the treatment was carried out.

On the whole, most authors consider that the number of complications after cytoreductive surgery combined with HIPEC is generally acceptable.

3.9 Conclusion

According to the literature reports, despite the improvement in survival rates of patients with pseudomyxoma and peritoneal mesothelioma achieved by cytoreductive surgery combined with intraperitoneal chemotherapy, there is still a number of unresolved issues such as, "What are the causes of developing pseudomyxoma in highly differentiated and benign lesions? What are their immunophenotypes? What is the role of intraperitoneal chemotherapy alone and in hyperthermia conditions, taking into account the fact that histological analysis of most removed tumors revealed a low proliferation index and the case history showed resistance to systemic chemotherapy? Are there any differences in the peritoneal tumor growth in relation to the differentiation grade of the primary tumor in case of pseudomyxoma? What is the effect of the treatment extended mode of the primary tumor on the following development of pseudomyxoma? Is it necessary to remove the intact parietal peritoneum with pseudomyxoma and mesothelioma, and, in that case, what is the optimal level of cytoreduction, given that a surgeon, as a rule, intends to perform the maximum cytoreduction? And can the intervention be considered optimal in case of a residual tumor of any size (CCR1)? What chemotherapy regimens should be considered rational? What should be done in case of relapses and continuing tumor growth?"

In addition, molecular, genetic, and immunologic characteristics of pseudomyxoma and mesothelioma present a very interesting and poorly studied problem, which may affect the disease prognosis.

Thus, a lot of controversial issues still remain topical after the analysis of literature data, which encourages further studying the problem.

References

1. Spiliotis J, Vaxevanidou A, Sergouniotis F, Lambropoulou E, Datsis A, Christopoulou A (2011) The role of cytoreductive surgery and hyperthermic intraperitoneal chemotherapy in the management of recurrent advanced ovarian cancer: a prospective study. J BUON 16(1):74–79
2. Mercier F, Bakrin N, Bartlett DL, Goere D, Quenet F, Dumont F, Heyd B (2018) Peritoneal carcinomatosis of rare ovarian origin treated by cytoreductive surgery and hyperthermic intraperitoneal chemotherapy: a multi-institutional Cohort from PSOGI and BIG-RENAPE. Ann Surg Oncol 25(6):1668–1675
3. Fournier M, Huchon C, Ngo C, Bensaid C, Bats AS, Combe P, le FrèreBelda MA, Fournier L, Berger A, Lecuru F (2018) Morbidity of rectosigmoid resection in cytoreductive surgery for ovarian cancer. risk factor analysis. Eur J Surg Oncol 3(18):748–798
4. Perrin M, Bentivegna E, Bonneau C, Uzan C, Leary A, Pautier P, Genestie C, Morice P, Gouy S (2018) Bevacizumab does not reduce the lymphocele rate in advanced ovarian cancer after complete cytoreductive surgery. Anticancer Res 38(4):2247–2252
5. Coccolini F, Campanati L, Catena F et al (2015) Hyperthermic intraperitoneal chemotherapy with cisplatin and paclitaxel in advanced ovarian cancer: a multicenter prospective observational study. J Gynecol Oncol 26:54–61
6. Chiva LM, Gonzalez-Martin A (2015) A critical appraisal of hyperthermic intraperitoneal chemotherapy (HIPEC) in the treatment of advanced and recurrent ovarian cancer. Gynecol Oncol 136:130–135
7. Halkia E, Spiliotis J, Sugarbaker P (2012) Diagnosis and management of peritoneal metastases from ovarian cancer. Gastroenterol Res Pract 2012:541842
8. Elias D, Honoré C, Dumont F, Ducreux M, Boige V, Malka D et al (2011) Results of systematic second look surgery plus HIPEC in asymptomatic patients presenting a high risk of developing colorectal peritoneal carcinomatosis. Ann Surg 254:289–293
9. Elias D, Goéré D, Dumont F, Honoré C, Dartigues P, Stoclin A et al (2014) Role of hyperthermic intraoperative peritoneal chemotherapy in the management of peritoneal metastases. Eur J Cancer 50:332–340
10. Mirnezami R, Moran BJ, Harvey K, Cecil T, Chandrakumaran K, Carr N et al (2014) Cytoreductive surgery and intraperitoneal chemotherapy for colorectal peritoneal metastases. World J Gastroenterol 20(38):14018–14032
11. Huang JY, Xu YY, Sun Z, Zhu Z, Song YX, Guo PT et al (2012) Comparison different methods of intraoperative and intraperitoneal chemotherapy for patients with gastric cancer: a meta-analysis. Asian Pac J Cancer Prev 13:4379–4385
12. Sun J, Song Y, Wang Z, Gao P, Chen X, Xu Y et al (2012) Benefits of hyperthermic intraperitoneal chemotherapy for patients with serosal invasion in gastric cancer: a meta-analysis of the randomized controlled trials. BMC Cancer 12:526
13. Sugarbaker PH (1998) Management of peritoneal surface malignancy using intraperitoneal chemotherapy and cytoreductive surger. Ludann Company, Michigan
14. Sugarbaker PH (1995) Peritonectomy procedures. Ann Surg 221:29–42
15. Shen P, Levine EA, Hall J et al (2003) Factors predicting survival after Intraperitoneal Hyprthermic Chemotherapy with mytomycin C after cytoreductive surgery for pts with peritoneal carcinomatosis. Arch Surg 138:26–33
16. Sugarbaker PH, Yonemura Y (2000) Clinical pathway for the management of resectable gastric cancer with peritoneal seeding: best palliation with a ray of hope for cure. Oncology 58:96–107
17. Beaujard AC, Glehen O, Caillot JL et al (2000) Intraperitoneal chemohyperthermia with mitomycin C for digestive tract cancer patients with peritoneal carcinomatosis. Cancer 88:2512–2519

18. Fujimoto S, Takahashi M, Kobayashi K et al (1992) Cytohistologic assessment of antitumor effects of intraperitoneal hyperthermic perfusion with mitomycin C for patients peritoneal metastasis. Cancer 70:2754–2760
19. Sugarbaker PH, Graves T, DeBruijn EA et al (1990) Rationale for early postoperative intraperitoneal chemotherapy (EPIC) in patients with advanced gastrointestinal cancer. Cancer Res 50:5790–5794
20. Sugarbaker PH, Sweatman TW, Graves T et al (1991) Early postoperative intraperitoneal adriamycin: pharmacologic studies and a preliminary clinical report. Reg Cancer Treat 4:127–131
21. Weisberger AS, Levine B, Storaasli JP (1955) Use of nitrogen mustard in treatment of serous effusions of neoplastic origin. J Am Med Assoc 159:1704–1707
22. Hagiwara A, Takahashi T, Sawai K et al (1993) Clinical trials with intraperitoneal cisplatin microspheres for malignant ascites – a pilot study. AntiCancer–Drug–Des 8(6):463–470
23. Ng EK, Chan AC, Lee WH, et al (1999) Prospective randomized trial of intraperitoneal charcoal–adsorbed mitomycin–C as an adjuvant to resectable T3 distal gastric cancer. 3-rd international gastric cancer congress. Seoul, Apr 27–30, p 102
24. Ohgaki M, Imanishi T, Ohyama T et al (1994) The prevention of peritoneal dissemination of gastric cancer with intraperitoneal activated carbon particles absorbing mitomycin C. Gan To Kagaku Ryoho 21(13):2320–2322
25. Kurita A, Takashima S, Takayama T, Doihara Y (1994) Intraperitoneal chemotherapy for gastric carcinoma combined with peritoneal dissemination by intraperitoneal catheter with a subcutaneous reservoir. JpnJCancer–Chemother 21(14):2439–2444
26. Ohta K, Ohyama S, Takahashi T, Nakajima T (1999) Usefulness of intraperitoneal administration of cisplatin using a reservoir for advanced gastric cancer complicated by peritoneal dissemination. 3-rd international gastric cancer congress. Seoul, Apr 27–30, p 98
27. Roviello F (2018) The role of HIPEC in gastric cancer. Eur J Cancer 92(Suppl 2):4–5
28. Yu W, Whang I, Chung HY, Averbach A, Sugarbaker PH (2001) Indication or early postoperative intraperitoneal chemotherapy of advanced gastric cancer: results of a prospective randomized trial. World J Surg 25(8):985–990
29. Yoo CH, Noh SH, Shin DW, et al (1999) Early postoperative intraperitoneal chemotherapy (EPIC) for advanced gastric cancer. Proceeding of the 3-rd international gastric cancer congress. Seoul, Apr 27–30, p 103
30. Nomura E, Niki M, Fujii K, et al (2001) Efficacy of intraperitoneal and intravenous chemotherapy and upper abdominal evisceration for advanced gastric cancer. 4-th international gastric cancer congress. New York. Apr 29–May 2, p 438
31. Ruth S, Mathot RA, Sparidans RW et al (2004) Population pharmacokinetics and pharmacodynamics of mitomycin during intraoperative hyperthermic intraperitoneal chemotherapy. Clin Armacokinet 43:131–143
32. Sticca RP, Dach BW (2003) Rationale for hyperthermia with intraoperative intraperitoneal chemotherapy agents. Surg Oncol Clin N Am 12:689–701
33. Oleson JR, Calderwood SK, Coughlin CT et al (1988) Biological and clinical aspects of hyperthermia in cancer therapy. Am J Clin Oncol 11:368–380
34. Issels RD (2008) Hyperthermia adds to chemotherapy. Eur J Cancer 44:2546–2554
35. Spratt JS, Adcock RA, Muskovin M et al (1980) Clinical delivery system for intraperitoneal hyperthermic chemotherapy. Cancer Res 40:256–260
36. Elias D, Bonnay M, Puizillou JM et al (2002) Heated intra-operative intraperitoneal oxaliplatin after complete resection of peritoneal carcinomatosis: pharmacokinetics and tissue distribution. Ann Oncol 13:267–272
37. Sugarbaker PH, Stuart OA, Carmignani CP (2006) Pharmacokinetic changes induced by the volume of chemotherapy solution in patients treated with hyperthermic intraperitoneal mito mycin C. Cancer Chemother Pharmacol 57:703–708
38. Torres IJ, Litterst CL, Guarino AM (1978) Transport of model compounds across the peritoneal membrane in the rat. Pharmacology 17:330–340

39. Groose E, Walker L, Masters JR (1986) The influence of osmolarity on drug cytotoxicity in vitro. Br J Cancer 54:181
40. Kondo A, Maeta M, Oka A et al (1996) Hypotonic intraperitoneal cisplatin chemotherapy for peritoneal carcinomatosis in mice. Br J Cancer 73:1166–1170
41. Tsujitani S, Oka A, Kondo A et al (1999) Administration in a hypotonic solution is preferable to dose escalation in intraperitoneal cisplatin chemotherapy for peritoneal carcinomatosis in rats. Oncology 57:77–82
42. Elias D, AEl O, Bonnay M et al (2002) Human pharmacokinetic study of heated intraperitoneal oxaliplatin in increasingly hypotonic solutions after complete resection of peritoneal carcinomatosis. Oncology 63:346–352
43. Pestieau SR, Schnake KJ, Stuart OA et al (2001) Impact of carrier solutions on pharmacokinetics of intraperitoneal chemotherapy. Cancer Chemother Pharmacol 47:269–276
44. Litterst CL, Torres IJ, Arnold S et al (1982) Adsorption of antineoplastic drugs following large-volume ip administration torats. Cancer Treat Rep 66:147–155
45. McArdle CS, Kerr DJ, O'Gorman P et al (1994) Pharmacokinetic study of 5-fluorouracil in a novel dialysate solution: a long-term intraperitoneal treatment approach for advanced colorectal carcinoma. Br J Cancer 70:762–766
46. Smeenk RM, Verwaal VJ, Zoetmulder FA (2006) Toxicity and mortality of cytoreduction and intraoperative hyperthermic intraperitoneal chemotherapy in pseudomyxoma peritonei–a report of 103 procedures. Eur J Surg Oncol 32:186–190
47. Shido A, Ohmura S, Yamamoto K et al (2000) Does hyperthermia induce peritoneal damage in continuous hyperthermic peritoneal perfusion? World J Surg 24:507–511
48. Zeamari S, Floot B, Van der Vange N et al (2003) Pharmacokinetics and pharmacodynamics of cisplatin after intraoperative hyperthermic intraperitoneal chemoperfusion (HIPEC). Anticancer Res 23:1643–1648
49. Moran BJ, Mukherjee A, Sexton R (2006) Operability and early outcome in 100 consecutive laparotomies for peritoneal malignancy. Br J Surg 93:100–104
50. Glehen O, Cotte E, Brigand C et al (2006) Therapeutic innovations in the management of peritoneal carcinomatosis from digestive origin: cytoreductive surgery and intraperitoneal chemotherapy. Rev Med Int 27:382–391
51. Elias D, Raynard B, Boige V et al (2005) Impact of the extent and duration of cytoreductive surgery on postoperative hematological toxicity after intraperitoneal chemohyperthermia for peritoneal carcinomatosis. J Surg Oncol 90:220–225
52. Kusamura S, Dominique E, Baratti D et al (2008) Drugs, carrier solutions and temperature in hyperthermic intraperitoneal chemotherapy. J Surg Oncol 98:247–252
53. Cravioto-Villanueva A, Cavazos M, Luna-Perez P, Martinez-Gomez H, Ramirez ML, Solorzano J et al (2016) Cytoreductive surgery with hyperthermic intraperitoneal chemotherapy (HIPEC) delivered via a modified perfusion system for peritoneal carcinomatosis of colorectal origin. Surg Today 46(8):979–984
54. Tyulyandin SA (2001) Chemotherapy for stomach cancer. Pract Oncol 7:44–51
55. Miner TJ, Shia J, Jaques DP, Klimstra DS, Brennan MF, Coit DG (2005) Long-term survival following treatment of pseudomyxoma peritonei: an analysis of surgical therapy. Ann Surg 241:300–308
56. Chua TC, Moran BJ, Sugarbaker PH, Levine EA, Glehen O, Gilly FN et al (2012) Early- and long-term outcome data of patients with pseudomxyoma perontonei from appendiceal origin treated by a strategy of cytoreductive surgery and hyperthermic intraperitoneal chemotherapy. J Clin Oncol 30:2449–2456
57. Glehen O, Mohamed F, Sugarbaker PH (2004 Aug) Incomplete cytoreduction in 174 patients with peritoneal carcinomatosis from appendiceal malignancy. Surgical Department, Centre Hospitalo-Universitaire Lyon Sud, Pierre Bénite, France. Ann Surg 240(2):278–285
58. Elias D, Gilly F, Quenet F, Bereder JM, Sidéris L, Mansvelt B et al (2010) Pseudomyxoma peritonei: a French multicentric study of 301 patients treated with cytoreductive surgery and intraperitoneal chemotherapy; Association Française de Chirurgie. Eur J Surg Oncol 36(5):7

59. Gough DB, Donohue JH, Schutt AJ et al (1994) Pseudomyxoma peritonei. Long term patient survival with an aggressive regional approach. Ann Surg 219:112–119
60. Glehen O, Gilly FN, Bereder JM, Quenet F, Sideris L, Mansvelt B et al (2010) Toward curative treatment of peritoneal carcinomatosis from nonovarian originby cytoreductive surgery combined with perioperative intraperitoneal chemotherapy a multi-institutional study of 1290 patients. Cancer 116(24):5608–5618
61. Loungnarath R, Causeret S, Bossard N, Faheez M, Sayag Beaujard AC, Brigand C, al e (2005) Cytoreductive surgery with intraperitoneal chemohyperthermia for the treatment of pseudomyxoma peritonei: a prospective study. Dis Colon Rectum 48:1372–1379
62. Wheeler BR, Reddy SK, Kenwright D, Keating JP (2014) Treating pseudomyxoma peritonei without heated intraperitoneal chemotherapy. N Z Med J 127(1389):31–39
63. Sridhar K, Doria R, Raub W, Thurer R, Saldana M (1992) New strategies are needed in diffuse malignant mesothelioma. Cancer 70:2969–2979
64. Antman K, Shemin R, Ryan L et al (1988) Malignant mesothelioma: prognostic variables in a registry of 180 patients, the Dana-Farber Cancer Institute and Brigham and Women's Hospital experience over two decades, 1965–1985. J Clin Oncol 6:147–153
65. Piccigallo E, Jeffers L, Reddy R, Caldironi M, Parenti A, Schiff E (1988) Malignant peritoneal mesothelioma. A clinical and laparoscopic study of ten cases. Dig Dis Sci 5:633–639
66. van Gelder T, Hoogsteden H, Versnel M, de Beer P, Vandenbroucke J, Planteydt H (1989) Malignant peritoneal mesothelioma: a series of 19 cases. Digestion 43:222–227
67. Antman KH, Pomfret EA, Aisner J, MacIntyre J, Osteen RT, Greenberger JS (1983) Peritoneal mesothelioma: natural history and response to chemotherapy. J Clin Oncol 1:386–391
68. Garcia-Carbonero R, Paz-Ares L (2006) Systemic chemotherapy in the management of malignant peritoneal mesothelioma. Eur J Surg Oncol 32:676–681
69. Turner K, Varghese S, Alexander HR (2012) Current concepts in the evaluation and treatment of patients with diffuse malignant peritoneal mesothelioma. J Natl Compr Cancer Netw 10(1):49–57
70. Langer CJ, Rosenblum N, Hogan M, Nash S, Bagchi P, LaCreta FP et al (1993) Intraperitoneal cisplatin and etoposide in peritoneal mesothelioma: favorable outcome with a multimodality approach. Cancer Chemother Pharmacol 32:204–208
71. Markman M, Kelsen D (1992) Efficacy of cisplatin-based intraperitoneal chemotherapy as treatment of malignant peritoneal mesothelioma. J Cancer Res Clin Oncol 118:547–550
72. Manzini V, Recchia L, Cafferata M, Porta C, Siena S, Giannetta L et al (2010) Malignant peritoneal mesothelioma: a multicenter study on 81 cases. Ann Oncol 21:348–353
73. Blackham AU, Shen P, Stewart JH, Russel GB, Levine EA (2010) Cytoreductive surgery with intraperitoneal chemotherapy for malignant peritoneal mesothelioma: mitomycin vs. cisplatin. Ann Surg Oncol 17:2720–2727
74. Yan TD, Deraco M, Baratti D, Kusamura S, Elias D, Glehen O et al (2009) Cytoreductive surgery and hyperthermic intraperitoneal chemotherapy for malignant peritoneal mesothelioma: multi-institutional experience. J Clin Oncol 27(36):6237–6242
75. Baratti D, Kusamura S, Nonaka D, Cabras AD, Laterza B, Deraco M (2009) Pseudomyxoma peritonei. Ann Surg 249(2):243–249
76. Kluger MD, Taub RN, Hesdorffer M, Jin Z, Chabot JA (2010) Two-stage operative cytoreduction and intraperitoneal chemotherapy for diffuse malignant peritoneal mesothelioma: operative morbidity and mortality in phase I and II trials. Eur J Surg Oncol (EJSO) 36(10):997–1003
77. Chua TC, Yan TD, Morris DL (2009) Outcomes of cytoreductive surgery and hyperthermic intraperitoneal chemotherapy for peritoneal mesothelioma: the Australian experience. J Surg Oncol 99(2):109–113
78. Robella VM, Mellano A et al (2014) Treatment of diffuse malignant peritoneal mesothelioma (DMPM) by cytoreductive surgery and HIPEC. Minerva Chir 69:9–15
79. Magge D, Zenati MS, Austin F, Mavanur A, Sathaiah M, Ramalingam L, Jones H, Zureikat AH, Holtzman M, Ahrendt S, Pingpank J, Zeh HJ, Bartlett DL, Choudry HA (2014)

Malignant peritoneal mesothelioma: prognostic factors and oncologic outcome analysis. Ann Surg Oncol 21(4):1159–1165
80. Helm JH, Miura JT, Glenn JA, Marcus RK, Larrieux G, Jayakrishnan TT et al (2015) Cytoreductive surgery and hyperthermic intraperitoneal chemotherapy for malignant peritoneal mesothelioma: a systematic review and meta-analysis. Ann Surg Oncol 22(5):1686–1693
81. Moran BJ (2006) Decision-making and technical factors account for the learning curve in complex surgery. J Public Health (Oxf) 28:375–378
82. Smeenk RM, Verwaal VJ, Zoetmulder FA (2007) Learning curve of combined modality treatment in peritoneal surface disease. Br J Surg 94:1408–1414
83. Yan TD, Links M, Fransi S et al (2007) Learning curve for cytoreductive surgery and perioperative intraperitoneal chemotherapy for peritoneal surface malignancy a journey to becoming a nationally funded peritonectomy center. Ann Surg Oncol 14:2270–2280
84. Sugarbaker PH, Welch LS, Mohamed F et al (2003) A review of peritoneal mesothelioma at the Washington Cancer Institute. Surg Oncol Clin N Am 12:605–621
85. Park BJ, Alexander HR, Libutti SK et al (1999) Treatment of primary peritoneal mesothelioma by continuous hyperthermic peritoneal perfusion (CHPP). Ann Surg Oncol 6:582–590
86. Deraco M, Nonaka D, Baratti D et al (2006) Prognostic analysis of clinicopathologic factors in 49 patients with diffuse malignant peritoneal mesothelioma treated with cytoreductive surgery and intraperitoneal hyperthermic perfusion. Ann Surg Oncol 13:229–237
87. Yan TD, Yoo D, Sugarbaker P (2006) Significance of lymphnodemetastasisinpatientswithdiffusemalignantperitonealmesothelioma. Eur J Surg Oncol 32:948–953
88. Yan TD, Brun E, Carlos A et al (2007) Prognostic indicators for patients undergoing cytoreductive surgery and perioperative intraperitoneal chemotherapy for diffuse malignant peritoneal mesothelioma. Ann Surg Oncol 14:41–49
89. Nonaka D, Kusamura S, Baratti D et al (2005) Diffuse malignant mesothelioma of the peritoneum: a clinicopathological study of 35 patients treated locoregionally at a single institution. Cancer 104:2181–2188
90. Brigand C, Monneuse O, Mohamed F et al (2006) Malignant peritoneal mesothelioma treated by cytoreductive surgery and intraperitoneal chemohyperthermia: results of a prospective study. Ann Surg Oncol 13:405–412
91. Loggie BW, Fleming RA, McQuellon RP et al (2001) Prospective trial for the treatment of malignant peritoneal mesothelioma. Am Surg 67:999–1003
92. Yan TD, Popa E, Brun E et al (2006) Sex difference in diffuse malignant peritoneal mesothelioma. Br J Surg 93:1536–1542
93. López-Basave HN, Morales-Vásquez F, Ruiz Molina JM et al (2011) Morbidity and mortality of cytoreductive surgery with hyperthermic intraperitoneal chemotherapy: national cancer institute, Mexico city, Mexico. ISRN Oncol 2011:526384
94. Mohamed F, Moran BJ (2009) Morbidity and mortality with cytoreductive surgery and intraperitoneal chemotherapy. Cancer J 15:196–199
95. Feldman AL, Libutti SK, Pingpank JF et al (2003) Analysis of factors associated with outcome in patients with malignant peritoneal mesothelioma undergoing surgical debulking and intraperitoneal chemotherapy. J Clin Oncol 21:4560–4567
96. Kusamura S, Younan R, Baratti D et al (2006) Cytoreductive surgery followed by intraperitoneal hyperthermic perfusion in the treatment of peritoneal surface malignancies: analysis of morbidity and mortality in 209 cases treated with closed abdomen technique. Cancer 106:1144–1153
97. Dindo D, Demartines N, Clavien P-A (2004) Classification of surgical complications: a new proposal with evaluation in a cohort of 6336 patients and results of a survey. Ann Surg 240:205–213
98. Bozzetti F, Braga M, Gianotti L et al (2001) Postoperative enteral versus parenteral nutrition in malnourished patients with gastrointestinal cancer: a randomised multicentre trial. Lancet 358:1487–1492

99. Younan R, Kusamura S, Baratti D et al (2005) Bowel complications in 203 cases of peritoneal surface malignancies treated with peritonectomy and closed-technique intraperitoneal hyperthermic perfusion. Ann Surg Oncol 12:910–918
100. Roviello F, Marrelli D, Neri A et al (2006) Treatment of peritoneal carcinomatosis by cytoreductive surgery and intraperitoneal hyperthermic chemoperfusion (IHCP): postoperative outcome and risk factors for morbidity. World J Surg 30(11):2033–2040
101. Younan R, Kusamura S, Baratti D et al (2008) Morbidity, toxicity, and mortality classification systems in the local regional treatment of peritoneal surface malignancy. J Surg Oncol 98:253–257
102. van Leeuwen BL, Graf W, Pahlman L, Mahteme H (2008) Swedish experience with peritonectomy and HIPEC. HIPEC in peritoneal carcinomatosis. Ann Surg Oncol 15(3):745–753
103. Rufian S, Munoz-Casares F, Bricefio J et al (2006) Radical surgery- peritonectomy and intraoperative intraperitoneal chemotherapy for the treatment of peritoneal carcinomatosis in recurrent or primary ovarian cancer. Ann Surg Oncol 94:316–324
104. Gusani NJ, Cho SW, Colovos C, Seo S, Franko J, Richard SD, Edwards RP, Brown CK, Holtzman MP, Zeh HJ, Bartlett DL (2008) Aggressive surgical management of peritoneal carcinomatosis with low mortality in a high-volume tertiary cancer center. Ann Surg Oncol 15(3):754–763
105. Clemente-Gutiérrez U, Garza-Gangemi A, Trejo-Gómez G, Medina-Franco H (2015) Morbidity and mortality following cytoreductive surgery with hyperthermic intraperitoneal chemotherapy at a tertiary care center: initial experience. Rev Investig Clin 67:39–45

Chapter 4
Standardizing of Mesothelioma and Pseudomyxoma Care

Ranyell Matheus Spencer Sobreira Batista and Thales Paulo Batista

Abstract Cytoreductive surgery (CRS) plus hyperthermic intraperitoneal chemotherapy (HIPEC) has emerged as a major comprehensive treatment of peritoneal surface malignancies. This multimodal approach has proved to be an effective curative treatment or a salvage therapy for a number of patients suffering from peritoneal surface malignancies and is currently the standard of care for appendiceal epithelial neoplasms and Pseudomyxoma peritonei (PMP) syndrome as well as diffuse malignant peritoneal mesothelioma (DMPM). Unfortunately, practices of CRS/HIPEC are widely variable in terms of technical particularities and antimitotic agents, which have produced heterogeneous and no comparable results. Since no single technique has so far demonstrated its superiority over the others, standardization of such practices may enhance patient outcomes, improve care standards and produce homogeneous data that permits systematic comparisons across all centers that offer this procedure.

Keywords Hyperthermia, Induced · Peritoneal neoplasms · Appendiceal neoplasms · Neoplasms, Mesothelial

4.1 Introduction

Cytoreductive surgery (CRS) plus hyperthermic intraperitoneal chemotherapy (HIPEC) has emerged as a major comprehensive treatment of peritoneal surface malignancies, especially for mesothelioma and pseudomyxoma subtypes due their characteristics, which include being confined to the abdominopelvic cavity, rarely invade organs and no metastatic spread [1]. Furthermore, CRS-HIPEC has been proved to be the only effective curative treatment for these patients being considered

R. M. S. S. Batista (✉)
Department of Pelvic Surgery, AC Camargo Cancer Center, São Paulo, Brazil

T. P. Batista
Department of Surgery/Oncology, IMIP, Recife, Brazil

Department of Surgery, Federal University of Pernambuco, Recife, Brazil

© Springer Nature Switzerland AG 2019

M. V. Kiselevskiy et al. (eds.), *Malignant Mesothelioma and Pseudomyxoma*,
https://doi.org/10.1007/978-3-319-99510-6_4

for best supportive care therapies [2, 3], while nowadays it is considered the standard of care for mucinous appendiceal neoplasms /pseudomyxoma peritonei (PMP) syndrome as well as diffuse malignant peritoneal mesothelioma (DMPM) [4, 5].

To proceed, we must know the pathological and clinical aspects of both mesothelioma and mucinous appendage neoplasms. This is the first step and will guide all treatment of these pathologies. Aspects related to response to systemic therapy, patient performance data and hospital medical training are fundamental steps for a treatment of excellence. The involvement of a multidisciplinary team with experienced professionals is also recommended for all cases in which cytoreductive and hypertherapeutic intraperitoneal chemotherapy (CRS/HIPEC) surgery is planned, thus making a tumor board meeting necessary.

Although apparently simple, conceptualizing peritoneal carcinomatosis, in a striking way to the treatment of CRS / HIPEC, is not an easy task. There are variations of macroscopic intraoperative and histopathologic aspects that often dictate the course of treatment, which cannot be considered only by the presence or not of peritoneal dissemination. The type of primary tumor, the infiltration or not of lesions, the region of involvement and the amount of disseminated disease should be evaluated prior to the decision to perform the CRS/HIPEC procedure. Many studies have tried to solve this question, and thus far laparoscopy has proven to be the most efficient method for this purpose [6].

CRS associated with hyperthermic intraperitoneal chemotherapy (HIPEC) has its key principles in the assumption that surgery allows the reduction of peritoneal disease to a microscopic or minimal condition, associated with the use of chemotherapy with predominantly local action enhanced by the addition of heat [7, 8]. Some studies also reveal that hyperthermia can reduce the mechanisms of cellular resistance to cisplatin and induce an efficient anticancer immune response via exposure of cell surface heat shock proteins [8–10].

Even with critics referring to a single application of the drug, maintaining long-term catheters does not guarantee complete bathing of the peritoneal cavity by the appearance of adhesions [11, 12]. Despite the high doses applied, the size of the chemotherapeutic molecule is an impediment for an excessive amount to pass through the blood-peritoneal barrier, reducing the risk of systemic dissemination and toxicity [7, 13]. The fact is that the CRS-HIPEC procedure has been or at least may show to be able to both increase overall disease-free survival and to leave the patient free of chemotherapy cycles to control peritoneal disease.

In this chapter, we will explore all of these aspects, in addition to briefly describing some steps of the surgery itself. Ultimately we hope the reader will know when to indicate the procedure, who to indicate it for and whether there is a need for any perioperative treatment. In addition, we will show some special situations that are part of the surgical routine, such as the best course for a patient with carcinomatosis incidentally discovered during a diagnostic laparoscopy.

4.1.1 Histological Aspects

Correct assessment of the histopathological aspects is essential, not only for prognostic value but also for treatment orientation. In fact, low-grade mucinous appendiceal adenocarcinomas with peritoneal involvement have a unique clinical behavior with the progressive accumulation of non-invasive intraperitoneal mucinous acellular material, which corresponds to the clinical syndrome of pseudomyxoma peritonei [4, 5]. The clinical picture is, for the most part, very characteristic; however, in cases where there is doubt, or by institutional protocols, an immunohistochemical study can be done. Muc-2, MUC-5 AC, caudal-related homeobox (CDX) -2, cytokeratin (CK) -7, and CK-20 proteins are investigated to differentiate adenocarcinomas from appendiceal mucinous neoplasms [14].

Historically one of the first studies that proposed to classify mucinous neoplasms of the appendix was published by Ronnett et al. [15]. The classification adopted was divided into three categories: (1) disseminated peritoneal adenomucinosis (DPAM), where there is abundant mucin and scant simple mucinous cells with little atypia and mitotic activity; (2) peritoneal mucinous carcinomatosis (PMCA), where the cellular and architectural features of carcinoma exist; (3) peritoneal mucinous carcinomatosis with intermediate or discordant features (PMCA-I/D), where intermediate features exist [16]. The prognosis is best for DPAM followed by PMCA-I/D and is worst for PMCA.

More studies have been done in this sense [17, 18] until most recently, the Peritoneal Surface Oncology Group International (PSOGI) [19] proposed a definition more practical and reproducible with two new pathological categories, namely AC and SRC-PMP, identifying two subsets of patients with favorable and exceedingly dismal prognosis, respectively [20]. However, it remains unclear whether the PSOGI classification might provide better prognostic stratification than the current The American Joint Committee on Cancer Classification 8th Edition [21]. In relation to the previous edition [22], there was the addition of the category *in situ* low-grade appendiceal mucinous neoplasm (LAMN) that has not penetrated the muscularis mucosae itself. Moreover, involvement of the subserosa and beyond is assigned the T3 or T4 category, as other invasive carcinomas.

4.1.2 Patient Selection

Selecting the patient well by observing both clinical and disease aspects is the initial start for treatment. There is no point in the disease being resectable if the patient cannot support the procedure, as this procedure cannot be offered to a patient with an impediment to performance due to its morbidity and mortality rates. This clinical anatomy evaluation should be continuous since the patient may change performance during various stages of treatment.

The patient must be carefully examined during the preoperative investigation, in addition to the request of cardiopulmonary evaluations (echocardiogram and lung function test), renal tests (creatinine clearance and serum creatinine) and liver and nutritional function tests (BMI, sarcopenia and albumin serum). There is also an overall consensus that patients who fit the criteria for a major comprehensive oncological approach such as CRS/HIPEC are those patients with ASA I-II, performance status of 0–2, with no limiting comorbidities and aged lower than 65–70 years [6, 23, 24].

The assessment of the amount of disease can also be performed preoperatively. Assessing the preoperative amount of disease is a difficult task since small lesions are not easily seen by imaging methods. Infiltrative aspects that affect a large part of the small intestine, hepatic hilum or pelvis that require very large procedures, may not indicate HIPEC or place the patient at a level of multiple surgeries. As a result, computed tomography, and if necessary, FDG-PET, magnetic resonance imaging or laparoscopic exploration, have been used with suboptimal accuracy [6, 25]. Although they are also considered in the preoperative evaluation, tumor markers are used more in postoperative follow-up [26].

Despite this effort, the calculation of tumor dissemination by the peritoneum is best evaluated by exploratory laparotomy, which often makes the decision to follow CRS-HIPEC an intraoperative act. This calculation is performed and estimated by the peritoneal cancer index (PCI) [27, 28], which, in addition to having prognostic value, is directly related to the success of the surgery, in what is referred to as complete cytoreduction or CC0 [27]. In practical terms, there is only benefit in HIPEC for the patients in which it was possible to undergo CC0 or CC1 surgeries.

Additionally, the distribution of peritoneal diffusion in the abdomen constitutes a limitation for performing CRS [6]. In these settings, the most frequent contraindications for CRS/HIPEC are extra-abdominal metastasis, massive involvement of the small bowel and its mesentery, hepatic pedicle and gastro-hepatic ligament, gross retroperitoneal lymph node involvement, and ureteral or biliary obstruction, whereas a restrictive cut-off value for PCI (i.e., PCI >20) also should not be applied as an absolute exclusion criterion for CRS/HIPEC suffering of PMP [6, 29, 30].

4.1.3 Perioperative Oncological Management

Perioperative oncological management involving systemic therapies for appendicular mucinous neoplasia is not clearly supported by prospective trials, only by data from experienced centers [31]. For instance, neoadjuvant chemotherapy for patients with DMPM did not have a better OS and was not associated with completeness of cytoreduction [31]. Furthermore, neoadjuvant chemotherapy had a negative impact over the survival for those who underwent CRS-HIPEC with curative intent. Conversely, adjuvant chemotherapy may delay recurrence and improve survival [32].

Patients often spend months and even years receiving chemotherapy before arriving at a referral center. The hypothesis that mucinous appendix neoplasia has a very low proliferative index reinforces the fact that it does not respond well to chemotherapy and this delay in being treated by experienced professionals is a fact of negative impact on survival. Therefore, the use of neoadjuvant or preoperative chemotherapy may be related to worse survival. Another hypothesis is that, usually, if neoadjuvant is indicated for patients with a large volume of disease under preoperative evaluation, namely, cases with very high PCI, it is already categorized as worse prognosis.

The fact is that the main modality of treatment is CRS plus HIPEC upfront and it should be considered the standard approach for DMPM, while waiting for a stronger level of scientific evidence [4, 32, 33]. Systemic chemotherapy should be administered principally in patients with recurrent disease or at a high risk for recurrence, and in those who are not appropriate candidates for aggressive surgery or who were not optimally debulked [18, 34]. However, in a subgroup analysis, patients with histological types of worse prognosis, such as the presence of signet ring cell and adenocarcinoid histomorphology, may benefit from the use of preoperative chemotherapy [35–37]. Although this topic is quite controversial, preoperative systemic chemotherapy appears to improve the prognosis of patients with signet ring cell histology [22]. In summary, the use of preoperative fluoropyrimidine-based systemic chemotherapy should be considered for high-grade peritoneal metastasis from appendiceal adenocarcinoma with signet ring cell histology and moderate to high PCI scores [22, 35].

Finally, regarding the use of early postoperative intraperitoneal chemotherapy (EPIC) in combination with CRS/HIPEC, our proposal of standardized procedures is not to routinely deliver EPIC for either PMP/appendiceal tumors or DMPM, since this additional procedure is associated with an increased rate of complications and adds no clear benefit in terms of survival [5, 11, 12] whereas HIPEC-alone protocols are much simpler for the patient, surgeon, and nursing care [11]. As previously reported, the use of EPIC did not translate to better survival outcomes in the largest surgical series exploring CRS/HIPEC for the treatment of PMP/appendiceal tumors [18] or DMPM [4], which supports this view.

4.1.4 Technical Aspects

Sugarbaker pioneered the technical aspects of CRS-HIPEC, which is now the basis for the procedure [38–40]. However, there were changes and new techniques described starting from the 80s. There is still much to be studied and eventually modified over time [41].

Following a sequence of procedures, the initial step is the positioning of the patient. Extreme care should be taken, considering that they are long surgeries where the positioning is able to cause neurological or decubitus injuries. Needed is nursing care with anti-impact dressings, observing leggings and limbs so that there is no tensioning and allow the proper placement of retractors, anesthetic care with bladder and nasogastric probing, and the passage of central venous access catheters and intraoperative monitoring. The placement of an epidural catheter for postoperative pain control can also be adopted. Goal-guided anesthesia is the most recommended, in that it avoids the infusion of large volumes of saline solutions and hemodynamic indicators allow the anesthesiologist to anticipate intraoperative needs.

The cavity opening should be xifopubic with peritoneal exposure. For cases where a complete CRS is estimated, it is often preferable that the peritoneum be removed early only after accessing the intraperitoneal cavity, thus facilitating subsequent resection (Fig. 4.1a–c). After intraperitoneal assessment of resectability, the initiation of the procedure is very much at the discretion of the surgeon. Some prefer to start with the subdiaphragmatic upper abdomen, while others prefer to start in the most critical regions such as the hepatic hilum or even where a large resection like the pelvic region is estimated (Figs. 4.2, and 4.3) Some groups have even proposed two-time resection in cases of large tumor volume in a clinically at-risk patient [42].

After resection, a started point of discussion is performing HIPEC as a closed or open abdominal (coliseum) technique. While there are no convincing data favoring any technique [43–45], an advantage of the closed technique is that it is simpler and can reduce the risk of contamination [46] (Fig. 4.4). After the catheters have been placed, infusion of solution, usually a solution of 1.5% isotonic peritoneal dialysis dextrose [46] or without chloride (for HIPEC where oxaliplatin is used) [47]. After reaching the ideal intraperitoneal temperature, around 42 °C [48] the drug infusion

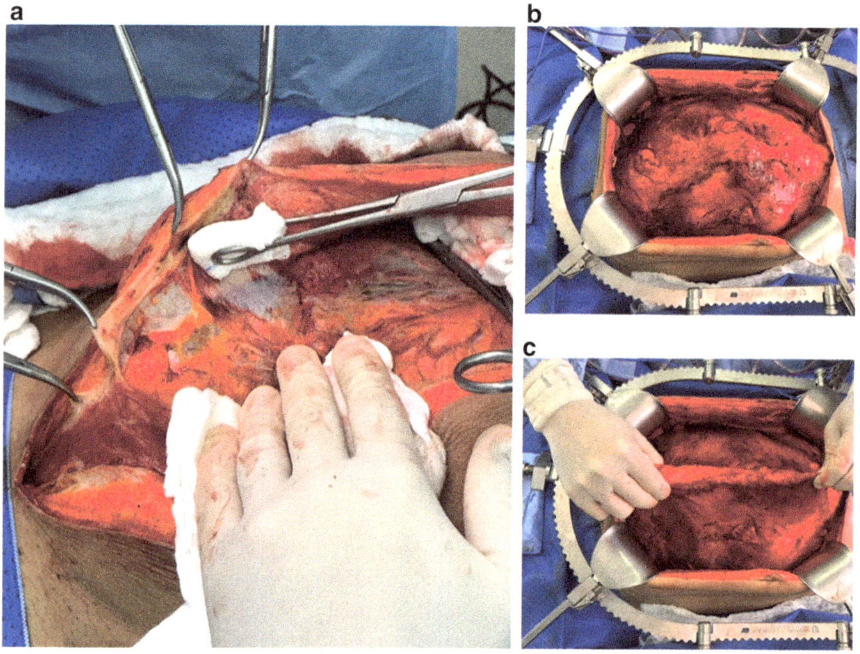

Fig. 4.1 Total anterior parietal peritonectomy. (**a**) The peritoneum is dissected away from the posterior rectus under retraction along the anterior abdominal wall. (**b**, **c**) Final view after the peritoneal stripping

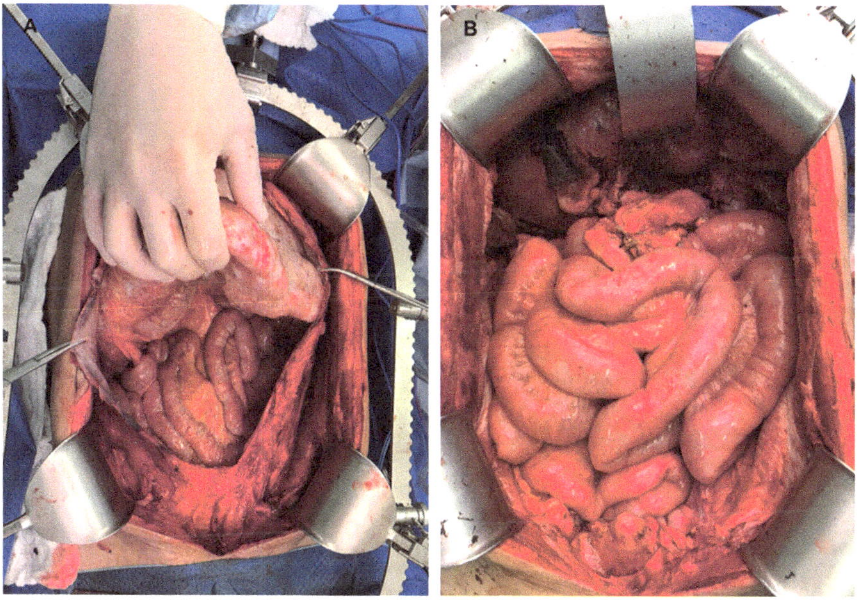

Fig. 4.2 Exposure of all the abdomen and visceral peritoneum. (**a**) Omental-cake retracted to explores the small bowel and its mesentery; (**b**) Result view after complete parietal and visceral peritonectomy

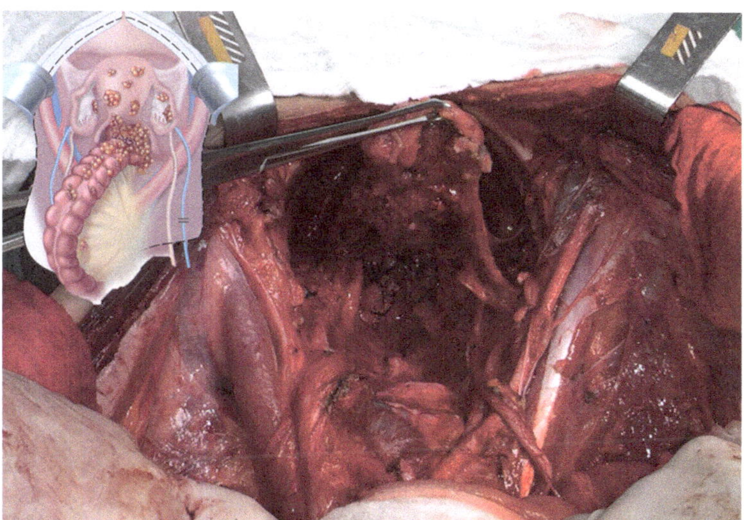

Fig. 4.3 Result view after complete pelvic peritonectomy, involving resections of rectosigmoid colon, cul-de-sac of Douglas and uterus/ovaries

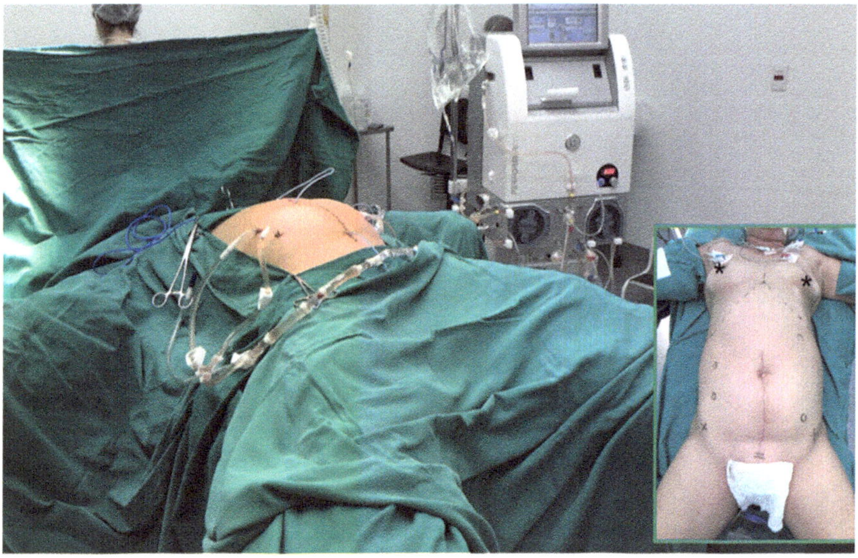

Fig. 4.4 Overall view of a HIPEC procedure performed as closed-technique

and the HIPEC time count is started. Despite variations, a total of 4 L including the chemotherapy solution is an option in view of uniformity with drug concentration, which does not mean that the total 4 L should be infused. The total volume infused is dictated by the clinical impression itself and by the measurement of the intra-abdominal pressure [49]. In regards of flow rate parameters, our proposal is that 300–500 mL/min should be applied during the "patient-filling phase" and thus increased to 700 mL/min during the "circulation" and "HIPEC" phases [50–52].

The time of bowel anastomoses varies. The argument is that, after HIPEC, there may be edema of loops which would make it difficult to perform anastomosis, in addition to the fact that there would be contact of the chemotherapy in exposed areas, which would not occur in patients with anastomosis performed previously. In fact, there is nothing to justify one or the other. A previous report from the fifth International Consensus Meeting on Peritoneal Surface Malignancies Treatment had favored the "after HIPEC" approach but the number (54%) is closely in the middle supporting neither [53]. However, in cases requiring an esophago-jejunal anastomosis after total gastrectomy, the best approach may be after HIPEC. This reduces the exposure of mediastinum to cardiotoxic drugs as cisplatin.

Diverting ileostomy is not routinely recommended and may be avoided at the surgeon's discretion after colorectal stapled anastomoses [54], especially because restoration of bowel continuity is often related to high rate of temporary stomas that will not be subsequently reversed [55] as well as to postoperative complication [56].

In addition to an experienced and skilled anesthesia team, modern and safe monitoring equipment should also be relied upon [57]. In these settings, one of the most recent reviews involving several aspects related to peri-, intra- and postoperative management of patients undergoing CRS/HIPEC has just been published by Raspé et al. [46] and summarizes the main understanding of that committee to improve perioperative care standards for the procedures. Intraoperative fluids management must be highlighted as a great paradigm change, which went from large volumes, to control guided by hemodynamic goals that often involves the use of early vasoactive drugs and volume restriction [58, 59].

Fast-track protocols are feasible in order to accelerate recovery, but should be carefully considered depending on surgical size and patient characteristics and risk factors [60–62]. An important aspect that should be remembered is that vaccines are performed in cases where splenectomy is planned during CRS-HIPEC. These patients should receive pneumococcal and influenza immunization at least 2 weeks prior or 14 or more days after procedures [63]; patients not previously immunized should also receive *Haemophilus influenza* type B and meningococcal group C conjugate vaccines [64, 65].

4.1.5 Right Colectomy During CRS–HIPEC Procedures

A right hemicolectomy is not routinely required in PMP resulting from mucinous appendiceal neoplasms at low risk of relapse or lymph node involvement [66, 67], as it does not confer a survival advantage in patients with mucinous carcinoma of the appendix and peritoneal seeding [68]. In the same study, the presence of lymph node metastases had no influence on prognosis. The authors suggested a more selective approach for LAMN. Routine right colon resection may be recommended only to an intestinal type of appendiceal cancer [53].

4.1.6 Perforated Mucocele: What to Do?

Frequently a dilemma exists after the resection of a mucocele in which the wall of the appendix has been perforated without any evidence of peritoneal surface malignancy involvement. The recommendations for those cases where outlined by Sugarbaker as the following: If the appendiceal specimen with perforation shows adenomucinosis, follow-up with computed tomography (CT) scans every 6 months for a duration of 5 years. With follow-up, if pseudomyxoma peritonei is clinically detected, its progression should be sufficiently indolent to allow a curative approach to the disease process [69]. However, if the appendiceal tumor shows mucinous adenocarcinoma in the appendix specimen, a second-look surgery should be recommended.

4.1.7 Mesothelioma Peritoneal

4.1.7.1 General Aspects

Mesothelioma is a tumor originating from the mesothelium of serous as pleura, peritoneum, pericardium and the vaginal tunic of the testicles. The incidence rate in USA, for both sex, peaked in the late 1980s and early 1990s, topping out in 1992 at 1.49 cases per 100,000. Nowadays, peritoneal mesothelioma accounts for about 10–20% of cases, corresponding to about 2500 new cases per year in the US and still very low survival, approximately 7–9% with life expectancy between 12–21 months [70]. More than 90% of cases occur in patients over 50 years of age, being more common in men, likely because the risk of greater exposure, the main cause of the disease, is asbestos [71, 72].

There are three histopathological subtypes or major variants of mesothelioma: sarcomatoid, epithelioid and biphasic. The sarcomatoid type has the worst prognosis with overall survival of 13 months at 5 years. Histologies with high Ki-67 are also considered poor responders (i.e., = 25% by immunohistochemical evaluation)77. The most common variant is the epithelioid type making up 50–70% of the cases. This variant is also the one that has the best prognosis with overall survival at 5 years of 55 months. There is also the biphasic variant that accounts for only 10% of the cases [71, 72].

Peritoneal mesothelioma (PM) has peculiar features where peritoneal dissemination is the main cause of morbidity and mortality. This diffusion may extend to the pleural cavity where it confers a worse prognosis. Only 6% of the lymph nodes are affected, but once suspected, this number can reach close to 30%. Distant metastases are uncommon and therefore the CRS-HIPEC strategy applies very well to such cases [74, 75]. One variant with an excellent prognosis is called multicystic. It mainly affects young or middle-aged women. Etiologic factors involved are: history of endometriosis, previous pelvic surgery and pelvic inflammatory disease. Although quite indolent, 50% of cases may recur [74, 76].

4.1.7.2 Treatment

There is no consensus as to the best treatment of peritoneal mesothelioma. Most of the clinical information available is retrospective data. In the past, most referral centers treated all cases with systemic chemotherapy and palliative surgery with or without total abdominal radiation therapy. With this strategy, the results were discouraging with median overall survival less than 12 months [77, 78].

As stated earlier, there are many reasons for CRS-HIPEC to have a role in this pathology. The fact that the tumor is most often confined to the peritoneal cavity with lesions that are often superficial and noninvasive provides complete cytoreduction or CC1 in more than 50% of cases [51]. However, this is not possible for all variants of mesothelioma, for example, for the sarcomatoid variant whose prognosis is worse. In these cases, only those well selected, namely without lymph node disease, low PID and responding to systemic chemotherapy are potential candidates for CRS-HIPEC [51].

Therefore, incorporating the histological variant into the other criteria that is, disease extent, age, degree of malnutrition and extraperitoneal involvement is a fundamental step both to indicate and to obtain the best results with CRS-HIPEC treatment [79]. Furthermore, patients with PM of histological biphasic or sarcomatoid subtype must not be considered for treatment with CRS/HIPEC4 as well as those tumors with high expression of Ki67 [73]. Similarly, patients with both Ki-67 > 10% and PCI > 17–20 are also unlikely to benefit from the procedure and should be considered for other treatment protocols [73, 80, 81]. Computed tomography findings such as the presence of epigastric mass greater than 5 cm in size and loss of normal architecture of the small intestine or mesentery nearly indicates the impossibility of complete cytoreduction [82].

One of the largest records of mesotheliomas treated with CRS-HIPEC was published in 2009. A total of 405 cases were evaluated. The vast majority of cases (79%) were of the epithelioid variant and the survival for cases where CC0/CC1 (46%) was achieved was 56 months, which is more than double for patients who were not treated in this way [83]. An interesting fact is noted by some groups where HIPEC performed with cisplatin was that it had a better prognosis in relation to other drugs, a fact that is not confirmed by other etiologies of carcinomatosis such as those of colorectal origin [84].

From the technical point of view, all the strategies mentioned in the cytoreductive part for pseudomyxoma can be adopted with the provision that in cases of mesothelioma, it seems that the resection of the entire peritoneum is better than only the affected parts. This more radical strategy can improve overall survival data [33].

4.1.8 Intraperitoneal Chemotherapy Schedules for DMPM and PMP

Even though several regimens of drugs for HIPEC procedures are available, one of the most common options for treatment of DMPM is cisplatin 100 mg/m^2 plus doxorubicin 15 mg/m^2 or carboplatin 800 mg/m^2, both for 60 min at 4 L of perfusate [52, 85]. For PMP and appendiceal tumors, some protocols include oxaliplatin 360 mg/m^2 for 30 min or cisplatin 100 mg/m^2 plus doxorubicin 15 mg/m^2 for 60 min, both at 4 L of perfusate [52]. These drug dosages should be reduced by about 30% for patients over the age of 60–70 years, patients previously exposed to multiple lines of systemic chemotherapy, patients who needed GM-CSF rescue for febrile neutropenia while on systemic chemotherapy patients who have received radiation therapy to bone-marrow bearing regions, and those who underwent extensive surgical cytoreduction due to high PCI scores [86, 87]. Accordingly, special attention is required for dose reduction of oxaliplatin to 200–250 mg/m^2 in these cases because of the increased risk of postoperative hemorrhagic complications compared with

Table 4.1 Chemotherapy (CT) scheme of HIPEC (closed technique) for pseudomixoma (PMP), appendiceal epithelial neoplasms and diffuse malignant peritoneal mesothelioma (DMPM)[a]

	Intraperitoneal chemotherapy schedules
	Oxaliplatin: 360 mg/m², 30 min at 4L of perfusate or;
PMP	CDDP: 100 mg/m² plus doxorubicin 15 mg/m², 60 min at 4L of perfusate, or;
	Mitomicin C[b]: 3 steps: 1st – 18 mg/m² at 1L of perfusate, plus 2st 8 mg/m² at 1/4L and 3st 8 mg/m² at 1/4L of perfusate.
DMPM	CDDP: 100 mg/m² plus doxorubicin 15 mg/m², 60 min at 4L of perfusate, or;
	Carboplatin 800 mg/m², 60 min at 1/4L of perfusate.

[a]Based on a proposal of Brazilian Society of Surgical Oncology (BSSO/SBCO) [90]
[b]First step is done at time 0, and the followers after 30 min each. Total time of perfusion of 90 min

HIPEC using other drugs [84]. For safety reasons, we point to dose limiting of 1000 mg/m² (or 200 mg/m²/L of perfusate) for carboplatin, total dose of 240 mg (or 45 mg/L of perfusate) for cisplatin, 15 mg/L of perfusate for doxorubicin, and 460 mg/m² for oxaliplatin [52, 85].

Controversies exist regarding whether mitomycin or oxaliplatin is better for DMPM. Despite some data suggest that MMC might be a better agent for HIPEC delivery than oxaliplatin in patients suffering of peritoneal carcinomatosis of colorectal origins with favorable histologies and low burden of disease (i.e., PSDSS I/II) [88], a large published study involving more than two thousand patients with PMP/appendiceal tumors treated by strategies of CRS/HIPEC in 16 specialized centers demonstrated no significant benefit in terms of overall survival for HIPEC with oxaliplatin vs. MMC (10y survival of 78% vs. 66%, respectively; differences not statistically significant) [18]. Similarly, due to the potential of increasing morbidity and complexity of procedures, the routine use of bidirectional oxaliplatin-based HIPEC regimens can increase risk; therefore, more convincing data needs to first be available [89]. A proposal of chemotherapy schema of HIPEC for pseudomixoma (PMP), appendiceal epithelial neoplasms and diffuse malignant peritoneal mesothelioma (DMPM) is showed in Table 4.1.

4.2 Conclusions

Cytoreductive surgery (CRS) plus hyperthermic intraperitoneal chemotherapy (HIPEC) is currently the standard of care for appendiceal epithelial neoplasms and *Pseudomyxoma peritonei* (PMP) syndrome as well as diffuse malignant peritoneal mesothelioma (DMPM). Herein, we have reviewed the practices of CRS/HIPEC and thus, and thus proposed standards for common technical aspects, patient selection, intraperitoneal chemotherapy schedules and perioperative oncological managements. The effort of producing an acceptable standardization to guide clinical practice concerning CRS/HIPEC procedures may contribute to may enhance patient outcomes, improve care standards and produce homogeneous data that permits systematic comparisons across all centers that offer this procedure.

References

1. La L (2015) Looking up: recent advances in understanding and treating peritoneal carcinomatosis. CA Cancer J Clin 65(4):284–298
2. Passot G, Vaudoyer D, Villeneuve L, Kepenekian V, Beaujard AC, Bakrin N et al (2016) What made hyperthermic intraperitoneal chemotherapy an effective curative treatment for peritoneal surface malignancy: a 25-year experience with 1125 procedures. J Surg Oncol 113(7):796–803
3. Levine EA, Stewart JH, Shen P, Russell GB, Loggie BL, Votanopoulos KI (2014) Intraperitoneal chemotherapy for peritoneal surface malignancy: experience with 1000 patients. J Am Coll Surg 218(4):573–585
4. Yan TD, Deraco M, Baratti D, Kusamura S, Elias D, Glehen O et al (2009) Cytoreductive surgery and hyperthermic intraperitoneal chemotherapy for malignant peritoneal mesothelioma: multi-institutional experience. J Clin Oncol 27(36):6237–6242
5. Helm JH, Miura JT, Glenn JA, Marcus RK, Larrieux G, Jayakrishnan TT et al (2015) Cytoreductive surgery and hyperthermic intraperitoneal chemotherapy for malignant peritoneal mesothelioma: a systematic review and meta-analysis. Ann Surg Oncol 22(5):1686–1693
6. Cotte E, Passot G, Gilly FN, Glehen O (2010) Selection of patients and staging of peritoneal surface malignancies. World J Gastrointest Oncol 2(1):31–35
7. Witkamp AJ, de Bree E, Van Goethem RZF (2001) Rationale and techniques of intra-operative hyperthermic intraperitoneal chemotherapy. Cancer Treat Rev 27(6):365–374
8. Hettinga JV, Konings AW, Kampinga HH (1997) Reduction of cellular cisplatin resistance by hyperthermia - a review. Int J Hyperth 13(5):439–457
9. Zunino B, Rubio-Patiño C, Villa E, Meynet O, Proics E, Cornille A et al (2016) Hyperthermic intraperitoneal chemotherapy leads to an anticancer immune response via exposure of cell surface heat shock protein 90. Oncogene 35(2):261–268
10. Pelz JO, Vetterlein M, Grimmig T, Kerscher AG, Moll E, Lazariotou M et al (2013) Hyperthermic intraperitoneal chemotherapy in patients with peritoneal carcinomatosis: role of heat shock proteins and dissecting effects of hyperthermia. Ann Surg Oncol 20(4):1105–1113
11. McConnell YJ, Mack LA, Francis WP, Ho T, Temple WJ (2013) HIPEC + EPIC versus HIPEC-alone: differences in major complications following cytoreduction surgery for peritoneal malignancy. J Surg Oncol 107(6):591–596
12. Lam JY, McConnell YJ, Rivard JD, Temple WJ, Mack LA (2015) Hyperthermic intraperitoneal chemotherapy + early postoperative intraperitoneal chemotherapy versus hyperthermic intraperitoneal chemotherapy alone: assessment of survival outcomes for colorectal and high-grade appendiceal peritoneal carcinomatosis. Am J Surg 210(3):424–430
13. Sugarbaker PH (2007) Laboratory and clinical basis for hyperthermia as a component of intracavitary chemotherapy. Int J Hyperth 23(5):431–442
14. Baiocchi G, Ferreira FO, Mantoan H, da Costa AA, Faloppa CC, Kumagai LY, de Mello CA, Takahashi RM, Nakagawa WT, Aguiar S Jr, Lopes A (2016) Hyperthermic intraperitoneal chemotherapy after secondary cytoreduction in epithelial ovarian cancer: a single- center comparative analysis. Ann Surg Oncol 23(4):1294–1301
15. Schomas DA, Miller RC, Donohue JH et al (1995) Intraperitoneal treatment for peritoneal mucinous carcinomatosis of appendiceal origin after operative management: long-term follow-up of the Mayo Clinic experience. Am J Pathol 19(12):588–595
16. Guo AT, Li YM, Wei LX (2012) Pseudomyxoma peritonei of 92 Chinese patients: Clinical characteristics, pathological classification and prognostic factors. World J Gastroenterol 18(24):3081–3088
17. Brendan MJ (2003) The etiology, clinical presentation and management of pseudomyxoma peritonei. Surg Oncol Clin N Am 12:585–603
18. Chua TC, Moran BJ, Sugarbaker PH, Levine EA, Glehen O, Gilly FN, Baratti D, Deraco M, Elias D, Sardi A, Liauw W, Yan TD, Barrios P, Gómez Portilla A, de Hingh IH, Ceelen WP, Pelz JO, Piso P, González-Moreno S, Van Der Speeten K (2012) Early- and long-term outcome data of patients with pseudomyxoma peritonei from appendiceal origin treated by a

strategy of cytoreductive surgery and hyperthermic intraperitoneal chemotherapy. J Clin Oncol 30(20):2449–2456
19. Carr NJ, Cecil TD, Mohamed F, Sobin LH, Sugarbaker PH, González-Moreno S, Taflampas P, Chapman S, Moran BJ (2016) Peritoneal Surface Oncology Group International. A consensus for classification and pathologic reporting of Pseudomyxoma Peritonei and associated appendiceal neoplasia: the results of the Peritoneal Surface Oncology Group International (PSOGI) Modified Delphi Process. Am J Surg Pathol 40(1):14–26
20. Cereser Junior CH, Giordani DSN, Weston AC, Pessini SA, Sugarbaker PH, Meinhardt Junior JG (2015) Ovarian cancer with carcinomatosis: a case report [abstract]. Eur J Surg Oncol 41(suppl 1):S202
21. Surgeons AC (2017) In: Amin MB, Edge S, Greene F et al (eds) AJCC cancer staging manual, 8th edn. Springer International Publishing, New York
22. Milovanov V, Sardi A, Studeman K, Nieroda C, Sittig M, Gushchin V (2016) The 7th edition of the AJCC staging classification correlates with biologic behavior of mucinous appendiceal tumor with peritoneal metastases treated with cytoreductive surgery and hyperthermic intraperitoneal chemotherapy (CRS/ HIPEC). Ann Surg Oncol 23(6):1928–1933
23. López-López V, Cascales-Campos PA, Schneider MA, Gil J, Gil E, Gomez-Hidalgo NR et al (2016) Cytoreductive surgery and hyperthermic intraperitoneal chemotherapy (HIPEC) in elderly patients. A systematic literature review. Surg Oncol 25(4):378–384
24. Alyami M, Lundberg P, Kepenekian V, Goéré D, Bereder JM, Msika S, Lorimier G, Quenet F, Ferron G, TEE al. B-R and RWG (2016) Cytoreductive surgery and hyperthermic intraperitoneal chemotherapy for peritoneal carcinomatosis in the elderly: a case- controlled, multicenter study. Ann Surg Oncol 23(suppl 5):737–745
25. Yan TD, Morris DL, Shigeki K, Dario B, Marcello D (2008) Preoperative investigations in the management of peritoneal surface malignancy with cytoreductive surgery and perioperative intraperitoneal chemotherapy: expert consensus statement. J Surg Oncol 98(4):224–227
26. Taflampas P, Dayal S, Chandrakumaran K, Mohamed F, Cecil TD, Moran BJ (2014) Preoperative tumour marker status predicts recurrence and survival after complete cytoreduction and hyperthermic intraperitoneal chemotherapy for appendiceal Pseudomyxoma Peritonei: analysis of 519 patients. Eur J Surg Oncol 40(5):551–520
27. González-Moreno S, Kusamura S, Baratti D, Deraco M (2008) Postoperative residual disease evaluation in the locoregional treatment of peritoneal surface malignancy. J Surg Oncol 98(4):237–241
28. Portilla AG, Shigeki K, Dario B, Marcello D (2008) The intraoperative staging systems in the management of peritoneal surface malignancy. J Surg Oncol 98(4):228–231
29. Esquivel J, Elias D, Baratti D, Kusamura S, Deraco M (2008) Consensus statement on the loco regional treatment of colorectal cancer with peritoneal dissemination. J Surg Oncol 98:263–267
30. Verwaal VJ, Kusamura S, Baratti D, Deraco M (2008) The eligibility for local-regional treatment of peritoneal surface malignancy. J Surg Oncol 98(4):220–223
31. Deraco M, Baratti D, Hutanu I, Bertuli R, Kusamura S (2013) The role of perioperative systemic chemotherapy in diffuse malignant peritoneal mesothelioma patients treated with cytoreductive surgery and hyperthermic intraperitoneal chemotherapy. Ann Surg Oncol 20(4):1093–1100
32. Kepenekian V, Elias D, Passot G, Mery E, Goere D, Delroeux D, Quenet F, Ferron G, Pezet D, Guilloit JM, Meeus P, Pocard M, Bereder JM, Abboud K, Arvieux C, Brigand C, Marchal F, Classe JM, Lorimier G, De Chaisemartin C, Guyon F, Mariani P, Ortega-Deballon GOFN for RPM (RENAPE) (2016) Diffuse malignant peritoneal mesothelioma: evaluation of systemic chemotherapy with comprehensive treatment through the RENAPE database: multi-institutional retrospective study. Eur J Cancer 65:69–79
33. Baratti D, Kusamura S, Cabras AD, Deraco M (2012) Cytoreductive surgery with selective versus complete parietal peritonectomy followed by hyperthermic intraperitoneal chemotherapy

in patients with diffuse malignant peritoneal mesothelioma: a controlled study. Ann Surg Oncol 19(5):1416–1424
34. Kindler HL (2013) Peritoneal mesothelioma: the site of origin matters. Am Soc Clin Oncol Educ Book 33:182
35. Cummins KA, Russell GB, Votanopoulos KI, Shen P, Stewart JH, Levine EA (2016) Peritoneal dissemination from high-grade appendiceal cancer treated with cytoreductive surgery (CRS) and hyperthermic intraperitoneal chemotherapy (HIPEC). J Gastrointest Oncol 7(1):3–9
36. Turner KM, Hanna NN, Zhu Y, Jain A, Kesmodel SB, Switzer RA et al (2013) Assessment of neoadjuvant chemotherapy on operative parameters and outcome in patients with peritoneal dissemination from high-grade appendiceal cancer. Ann Surg Oncol 20(4):1068–1073
37. Hemelandu C, Sugarbaker PH (2016) Clinicopathologic and prognostic features in patients with peritoneal metastasis from mucinous adenocarcinoma, adenocarcinoma with signet ring cells, and adenocarcinoid of the appendix treated with cytoreductive surgery and perioperative intraperitoneal chemotherapy. Ann Surg Oncol 23(5):1474–1480
38. Deraco M, Baratti D, Kusamura S, Laterza B, Balestra MR (2009) Surgical technique of parietal and visceral peritonectomy for peritoneal surface malignancies. J Surg Oncol 100(4):321–328
39. Sugarbaker PH (2013) Cytoreductive surgery using peritonectomy and visceral resections for peritoneal surface malignancy. Transl Gastrointest Cancer 2(2):54–74
40. Sugarbaker PH (1995) Peritonectomy procedures. Ann Surg 221(1):29–42
41. Spratt JS, Adcock RA, Muskovin M, Sherrill W, McKeown J (1980) Clinical delivery system for intraperitoneal hyperthermic chemotherapy. Cancer Res 40(2):256–260
42. Akaishi E, Teixeira F, Katayama M, Mizumoto N, Costa FP, Buzaid AC, Hoff PM (2009) Peritonectomy for peritoneal carcinomatosis: long-term outcomes from a single Brazilian institution. World J Surg 33(4):835–839
43. Rodríguez Silva C, Moreno Ruiz FJ, Bellido Estévez I, Carrasco Campos J, Titos García A, Ruiz López M et al (2017) Are there intra-operative hemodynamic differences between the Coliseum and closed HIPEC techniques in the treatment of peritoneal metastasis? A retrospective cohort study. World J Surg Oncol 15(1):51
44. Halkia E, Tsochrinis A, Vassiliadou DT, Pavlakou A, Vaxevanidou A, Datsis A et al (2015) Peritoneal carcinomatosis: intraoperative parameters in open (coliseum) versus closed abdomen HIPEC. Int J Surg Oncol 2015:610597
45. Facy O, Combier C, Poussier M, Magnin G, Ladoire S, Ghiringhelli F et al (2015) High pressure does not counterbalance the advantages of open techniques over closed techniques during heated intraperitoneal chemotherapy with oxaliplatin. Surgery 157(1):72–78
46. Raspé C, Flöther L, Schneider R, Bucher M, Piso P (2017) Best practice for perioperative management of patients with cytoreductive surgery and HIPEC. Eur J Surg Oncol 43(6):1013–1027
47. Mehta AM, Van den Hoven JM, Rosing H, Hillebrand MJ, Nuijen B, Huitema AD et al (2015) Stability of oxaliplatin in chloride-containing carrier solutions used in hyperthermic intraperitoneal chemotherapy. Int J Pharm 479(1):23–27
48. Schaaf L, van der Kuip H, Zopf W, Winter S, Münch M, Mürdter TE et al (2015) A temperature of 40 °C appears to be a critical threshold for potentiating cytotoxic chemotherapy in vitro and in peritoneal carcinomatosis patients undergoing HIPEC. Ann Surg Oncol 22(Suppl 3):S758–S765
49. Rettenmaier MA, Mendivil AA, Gray CM, Chapman AP, Stone MK, Tinnerman EJ et al (2015) Intra-abdominal temperature distribution during consolidation hyperthermic intraperitoneal chemotherapy with carboplatin in the treatment of advanced stage ovarian carcinoma. Int J Hyperth 31(4):396–402
50. Batista TP, Badiglian-Filho L, Leão CS (2016) Exploring flow rate selection in HIPEC procedures. Rev Col Bras Cir 43(6):476–479
51. Glehen O, Cotte E, Kusamura S, Deraco M, Baratti D, Passot G et al (2008) Hyperthermic intraperitoneal chemotherapy: nomenclature and modalities of perfusion. J Surg Oncol 98(4):242–246

52. Kusamura S, Dominique E, Baratti D, Younan R, Deraco M (2008) Drugs, carrier solutions and temperature in hyperthermic intraperitoneal chemotherapy. J Surg Oncol 98(4):247–252
53. Kusamura S, O'Dwyer ST, Baratti D, Younan RDM (2008) Technical aspects of cytoreductive surgery. J Surg Oncol 98(4):232–236
54. Sugarbaker H (2016) Avoiding diverting ileostomy in patients requiring complete pelvic peritonectomy. Ann Surg Oncol 23(5):1481–1485
55. Riss S, Chandrakumaran K, Dayal S, Cecil TD, Mohamed F, Moran BJ (2015) Risk of definitive stoma after surgery for peritoneal malignancy in 958 patients: comparative study between complete cytoreductive surgery and maximal tumor debulking. Eur J Surg Oncol 41(3):392–395
56. de Cuba EM, Verwaal VJ, de Hingh IH, van Mens LJ, Nienhuijs SW, Aalbers AG et al (2014) Morbidity associated with colostomy reversal after cytoreductive surgery and HIPEC. Ann Surg Oncol 21(3):883–890
57. Maciver AH, Al-Sukhni E, Esquivel J, Skitzki JJ, Kane JM, Francescutti FV (2017) Current delivery of hyperthermic intraperitoneal chemotherapy with cytoreductive surgery (CS/HIPEC) and perioperative practices: an international survey of high-volume surgeons. Ann Surg Oncol 24(4):923–930
58. Mavroudis C, Alevizos L, Stamou KM, Vogiatzaki T, Eleftheriadis S, Korakianitis O et al (2015) Hemodynamic monitoring during heated intraoperative intraperitoneal chemotherapy using the FloTrac/ Vigileo system. Int Surg 100(6):1033–1039
59. Colantonio L, Claroni C, Fabrizi L, Marcelli ME, Sofra M, Giannarelli D et al (2015) A randomized trial of goal directed vs. standard fluid therapy in cytoreductive surgery with hyperthermic intraperitoneal chemotherapy. J Gastrointest Surg 19(4):722–729
60. Glehen O, Osinsky D, Cotte E, Kwiatkowski F, Freyer G, Isaac S et al (2003) Intraperitoneal chemohyperthermia using a closed abdominal procedure and cytoreductive surgery for the treatment of peritoneal carcinomatosis: morbidity and mortality analysis of 216 consecutive procedures. Ann Surg Oncol 10(8):863–869
61. Cascales-Campos PA, Sánchez-Fuentes PA, Gil J, Gil E, López-López V, Rodriguez Gomez-Hidalgo N et al (2016) Effectiveness and failures of a fast track protocol after cytoreduction and hyperthermic intraoperative intraperitoneal chemotherapy in patients with peritoneal surface malignancies. Surg Oncol 25(4):349–354
62. Cascales Campos PA, Gil Martínez J, Galindo Fernández PJ, Gil Gómez E, Martínez Frutos IM, Parrilla Paricio P (2011) Perioperative fast track program in intraoperative hyperthermic intraperitoneal chemotherapy (HIPEC) after cytoreductive surgery in advanced ovarian cancer. Eur J Surg Oncol 37(6):543–548
63. Dagbert F, Thievenaz R, Decullier E, Bakrin N, Cotte E, Rousset P et al (2016) Splenectomy increases postoperative complications following cytoreductive surgery and hyperthermic intraperitoneal chemotherapy. Ann Surg Oncol 23(6):1980–1985
64. Moulis G, Lapeyre-Mestre M, Mahévas M, Montastruc JL, Sailler L (2015) Need for an improved vaccination rate in primary immune thrombocytopenia patients exposed to rituximab or splenectomy. A nationwide population-based study in France. Am J Hematol 90(4):301–305
65. Davies JM, Barnes R, Miligan D, FBC for S in HWP of the HT (2002) Update of guidelines for the prevention and treatment of infection in patients with an absent or dysfunctional spleen. Clin Med 2(5):440–443
66. Foster JM, Gupta PK, Carreau JH, Grotz TE, Blas JV, Gatalica Z et al (2012) Right hemicolectomy is not routinely indicated in pseudomyxoma peritonei. Am Surg 78(2):171–177
67. Sugarbaker PH (2017) When and when not to perform a right colon resection with mucinous appendiceal neoplasms. Ann Surg Oncol 24(3):729–732
68. González-Moreno S, Sugarbaker PH (2004) Right hemicolectomy does not confer a survival advantage in patients with mucinous carcinoma of the appendix and peritoneal seeding. Br J Surg 91(3):304–311
69. Sugarbaker PH (2006) New standard of care for appendiceal epithelial neoplasms and pseudomyxoma peritonei syndrome? Lancet Oncol 7(1):69–76

70. Surveillance, Epidemiology and End Results (2017) Mesothelioma recent trends in SEER incidence rates; 2000–2014. https://seer.cancer.gov/explorer/application.php?site=111&data_type=1&stat_type=2
71. Teta MJ, Mink PJ, Lau E, Sceurman BK, Foster ED (2008) US mesothelioma patterns 1973–2002: indicators of change and insights into background rates. Eur J Cancer Prev 17(6):525–534
72. Robinson BW, Lake RA (2005) Advances in malignant mesothelioma. N Engl J Med 353(15):1591–1603
73. Pillai K, Pourgholami MH, Chua TC, Morris DL (2015) Prognostic significance of Ki67 expression in malignant peritoneal mesothelioma. Am J Clin Oncol 38(4):388–394
74. Sugarbaker PH, Welch LS, Mohamed F, Glehen O (2003) A review of peritoneal mesothelioma at the Washington Cancer Institute. Surg Oncol Clin N Am 12(3):605–621
75. van der Bij S, Koffijberg H, Burgers JA, Baas P, van de Vijver MJ, de Mol BA, Moons KG (2012) Prognosis and prognostic factors of patients with mesothelioma: a population-based study. Br J Cancer 107(1):161–164
76. Takeshima Y, Amatya VJ, Kushitani K, Inai K (2008) A useful antibody panel for differential diagnosis between peritoneal mesothelioma and ovarian serous carcinoma in Japanese cases. Am J Clin Pathol 130(5):771–779
77. Eltabbakh GH, Piver MS, Hempling RE, Recio FO, Intengen ME (1999) Clinical picture, response to therapy, and survival of women with diffuse malignant peritoneal mesothelioma. J Surg Oncol 70:6–12
78. Antman KH, Pomfret EA, Aisner J, MacIntyre J, Osteen RT, Greenberger JS (1983) Peritoneal mesothelioma: natural history and response to chemotherapy. J Clin Oncol 1(6):386–391
79. Cao C, Yan TD, Deraco M, Elias D, Glehen O, Levine EA, Moran BJ (2012) Importance of gender in diffuse malignant peritoneal mesothelioma. Ann Oncol 23(6):1494–1498
80. Baratti D, Kusamura S, Cabras AD, Bertulli R, Hutanu I, Deraco M (2013) Diffuse malignant peritoneal mesothelioma: long-term survival with complete cytoreductive surgery followed by hyperthermic intraperitoneal chemotherapy (HIPEC). Eur J Cancer 49(15):3140–3148
81. Kusamura S, Torres Mesa PA, Cabras A, Baratti D, Deraco M (2016) The role of Ki-67 and pre-cytoreduction parameters in selecting diffuse malignant peritoneal mesothelioma (DMPM) patients for cytoreductive surgery (CRS) and hyperthermic intraperitoneal chemotherapy (HIPEC). Ann Surg Oncol 23(5):1468–1473
82. Yan TD, Haveric N, Carmignani CP, Chang D, Sugarbaker PH (2005) Abdominal computed tomography scans in the selection of patients with malignant peritoneal mesothelioma for comprehensive treatment with cytoreductive surgery and perioperative intraperitoneal chemotherapy. Cancer 103(4):839–849
83. Yan TD, Deraco M, Baratti D, Kusamura S, Elias D, Glehen O, Gilly F¸o N, Levine EA, Shen P, Mohamed F, Moran BJ, Morris DL, Chua TC, Piso P, Sugarbaker PH (2009) Cytoreductive surgery and hyperthermic intraperitoneal chemotherapy for malignant peritoneal mesothelioma: multi-institutional experience. J Clin Oncol 27(36):6237–6242
84. Blackham AU, Shen P, Stewart JH, Russell GB, Levine EA (2010) Cytoreductive surgery with intraperitoneal hyperthermic chemotherapy for malignant peritoneal mesothelioma: mitomycin versus cisplatin. Gastrointest Oncol 17(10):2720–2727
85. Shetty SJ, Bathla L, Govindarajan V, Thomas PLB (2014) Comparison of cytoreductive surgery and hyperthermic intraperitoneal chemotherapy with mitomycin or carboplatin for diffuse malignant peritoneal mesothelioma. Am Surg 80(4):348–352
86. González-Moreno S, González-Bayón LA, Ortega PG (2010) Hyperthermic intraperitoneal chemotherapy: rationale and technique. World J Gastrointest Oncol 2(2):68–75
87. Baratti D, Kusamura S, Laterza B, Balestra MR, Deraco M (2010) Early and long-term postoperative management following cytoreductive surgery and hyperthermic intraperitoneal chemotherapy. World J Gastrointest Oncol 2(1):36–43

88. Prada-Villaverde A, Esquivel J, Lowy AM, Markman M, Chua T, Pelz J et al (2014) The American society of peritoneal surface malignancies evaluation of HIPEC with Mitomycin C versus Oxaliplatin in 539 patients with colon cancer undergoing a complete cytoreductive surgery. J Surg Oncol 110(7):779–785
89. Quenet F, Goéré D, Mehta SS, Roca L, Dumont F, Hessissen M et al (2011) Results of two bi-institutional prospective studies using intraperitoneal oxaliplatin with or without irinotecan during HIPEC after cytoreductive surgery for colorectal carcinomatosis. Ann Surg 254(2):294–301
90. Batista TP, Sarmento BJQ, Loureiro JF, Petruzziello L, Santos CC et al (2017) A proposal of Brazilian society of surgical oncology (BSSO/SBCO) for standardizing cytoreductive surgery (CRS) plus hyperthermic intraperitoneal chemotherapy (HIPEC) procedures in Brazil: pseudomixoma peritonei, appendiceal tumors and malignant peritoneal mesothelioma. Rev Col Bras Cir 44(5):530–544

Chapter 5
Experimental Basis for Optimal Regimnes of Hyperthermic Peritoneal Chemotherapy

Natalia Yu. Anisimova, Irina Zh. Zhubina, Fedor V. Donenko, Julia I. Dolzhikova, Antonina V. Kshnaykina, and Mikhail V. Kiselevskiy

Abstract Temperature exposure reliably inhibits tumor cell potential for proliferation at the temperature of not less than 43 °C only. Temperature regimens recommended for clinical treatment (40–42 °C) have no significant impact on the viability of tumor cells. Tumor growth arrest in murine models was observed only in case of preliminary warming of inoculated cells at a temperature more than 42 °C. Heating tumor cells up to 39 °C and their incubation with anticancer drugs in the mean-effective concentrations enhanced tumor cell sensitivity towards cytotoxic action of activated lymphocytes.

Keywords Hyperthermia · Anticancer drugs · Cytotoxicity · Tumor cells · Effectors of antitumor immunity

5.1 Impact of Hyperthermia on Physiological Activity of Tumor and Non-Transformed Cells *In Vitro*

Over the last two decades new approaches have been developed for treatment of peritoneal carcinomatosis and these are called in general as "cytoreductive surgery in combination with intraperitoneal chemotherapy with hyperthermia". A number of authors consider such treatment as the standard therapy for pseudomyxoma peritonei, mesothelioma, and intraperitoneally disseminated ovarian cancer; however the effectiveness of this therapy is still a debatable issue [1, 2].

The idea of hyperthermic exposure is based on the following principles:

N. Y. Anisimova (✉) · I. Z. Zhubina · F. V. Donenko · J. I. Dolzhikova · A. V. Kshnaykina
M. V. Kiselevskiy
Laboratory of Cell Immunity, N.N. Blokhin National Medical Research Center, Moscow, Russia

© Springer Nature Switzerland AG 2019

M. V. Kiselevskiy et al. (eds.), *Malignant Mesothelioma and Pseudomyxoma*, https://doi.org/10.1007/978-3-319-99510-6_5

1. providing a high concentration of cytostatics at the site of the malignant process;
2. reduction of systemic toxicity;
3. modulation of anticancer drug actions.

Average temperatures of the solution for peritoneal perfusion, suggested by different authors, range from 39 to 45 °C. Therefore, one of the most important issues of intraperitoneal hyperthermia – defining an optimal temperature regimen that implies the highest tumor cytotoxicity associated with the minimum complications – remains unresolved. In clinical settings, though, it is difficult to achieve such parameters taking into account variable tissue heat conduction connected with specific vascularization [3–6]. On the whole, there are a number of unsolved problems and the major one is defining the most favorable temperature regimen of the highest tumor cytotoxicity and the minimum side effects. In this context we performed a research to analyze hyperthermia effect on the viability of tumor cells and non-transformed cells *in vitro* and *in vivo*.

The viability of K-562 cells (human myelogenous leukemia), MCF7 (breast cancer), SCOV3 (human ovarian cancer), Colon (human colorectal cancer), B16 (mouse melanoma), Ehrlich (mouse breast carcinoma), embryonic VERO (renal cells of African green monkey), CVC (endothelial cells of calf vessels), and LEC (embryo cow lung cells) cells was assessed after cultivation in the hyperthermia conditions. The cell suspension in culture medium RPMI-1640 was warmed for 2 h at the temperature of 41–50 °C (control cells – at 37 °C). The percentage of physiologically active cells in the cultures was determined by MTT Assay. To assess proliferative cell activity of the cell cultures, the test was repeated 2 days later (Tables 5.1 and 5.2, Figs. 5.1 and 5.2).

The results showed that reliable reduction of physiologically active cells as compared to that of control cells after heating for 2 h at temperatures below 45 °C was observed only in tumor cell K-562 (≤−29%), MCF7 (≤−34%) and SCOV3 at t = 46 °C (≤−38%), while similar effect on non-transformed cells was registered

Table 5.1 Change of tumor and non-transformed cell viability after warming (41–50 °C) in comparison with control (37 °C)

	Cell line					
Temperature, °C	K-562	MCF7	SCOV3	VERO	CVC	LEC
41	−2 ± 8	−3 ± 11	0 ± 16	0 ± 4	−12 ± 15	−5 ± 22
42	−2 ± 10	−4 ± 10	−7 ± 11	−5 ± 7	−16 ± 13	−8 ± 11
43	−4 ± 5	−3 ± 10	−10 ± 9	−4 ± 13	−24 ± 13	−10 ± 15
44	−25 ± 10	−28 ± 4	−23 ± 7	−18 ± 22	−25 ± 4	−20 ± 5
45	−27 ± 7*	−34 ± 3*	−30 ± 9	−25 ± 8	−28 ± 11	−22 ± 10
46	−34 ± 2*	−42 ± 5*	−38 ± 5*	−32 ± 10	−48 ± 19	−25 ± 16
47	−48 ± 11*	−56 ± 14*	−50 ± 5*	−57 ± 14*	−57 ± 21*	−30 ± 12
48	−66 ± 7*	−63 ± 5*	−66 ± 16*	−61 ± 14*	−71 ± 14*	−38 ± 8*
50	−74 ± 14*	−65 ± 20*	−83 ± 19*	−74 ± 24*	−84 ± 24*	−69 ± 16*

$p \leq 0.05$ vs control

Table 5.2 Change of tumor and non-transformed cell proliferation after warming (41–50 °C) in comparison with control (37 °C)

	Cell line					
Temperature, °C	K-562	MCF7	SCOV3	VERO	CVC	LEC
41	−3 ± 23	−2 ± 7	−15 ± 15	−16 ± 12	−22 ± 18	−3 ± 2
42	−4 ± 10	−3 ± 5	−23 ± 12	−14 ± 4	−24 ± 2	−24 ± 5
43	−11 ± 14	−20 ± 11	−27 ± 2*	−18 ± 5	−24 ± 4	−28 ± 9
44	−39 ± 10*	−42 ± 7*	−34 ± 7*	−25 ± 5	−38 ± 22	−30 ± 9
45	−42 ± 15*	−45 ± 5*	−50 ± 8*	−31 ± 10	−49 ± 11*	−44 ± 10*
46	−51 ± 11*	−79 ± 10*	−56 ± 16*	−38 ± 10*	−63 ± 4*	−42 ± 1*
47	−68 ± 20*	−90 ± 10*	−75 ± 10*	−42 ± 5*	−65 ± 11*	−46 ± 8*
48	−92 ± 8*	−98 ± 5*	−79 ± 11*	−64 ± 13*	−74 ± 12*	−64 ± 7*
50	−98 ± 2*	−100 ± 1*	−83 ± 17*	−77 ± 18*	−73	−89

$p \leq 0.05$ vs control

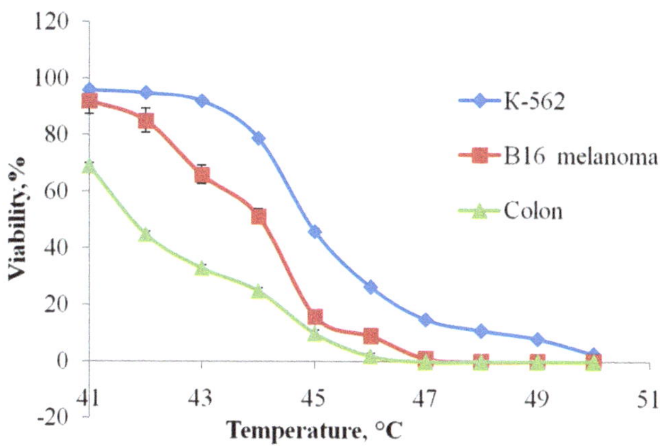

Fig. 5.1 Changes of viability of K-562, melanoma and Colon cell after hyperthermic exposure (for 2 h)

only at temperatures 47 °C (or higher) (VERO -≤−57%, CVC -≤−57%) and 48 °C (LEC-≤−38%).

Figure 5.1 demonstrates the similar reaction of human and animal cells to heating. The most labile cells were Colon cancer cells, the least – K-562 cells. The viability of Colon cells decreased by 50% after heating at 44 °C, B16 melanoma and K-562 –at 44 °C. However, the Fig. 5.2 shows that there remained visible proliferating Colon cells even after heating at a temperature of 44 °C for 2 h. Statistically significant inhibition of proliferative activity of the cells ($p \leq 0.01$) after 2-days' hyperthermic exposure was observed in the samples heated to 44 °C and higher (tumor cells) or 45 °C and higher (non-transformed embryonic cells).

A significant decrease of Ehrlich cells proliferative activity was observed only after exposure to the temperatures of 43 °C and higher (Fig. 5.3).

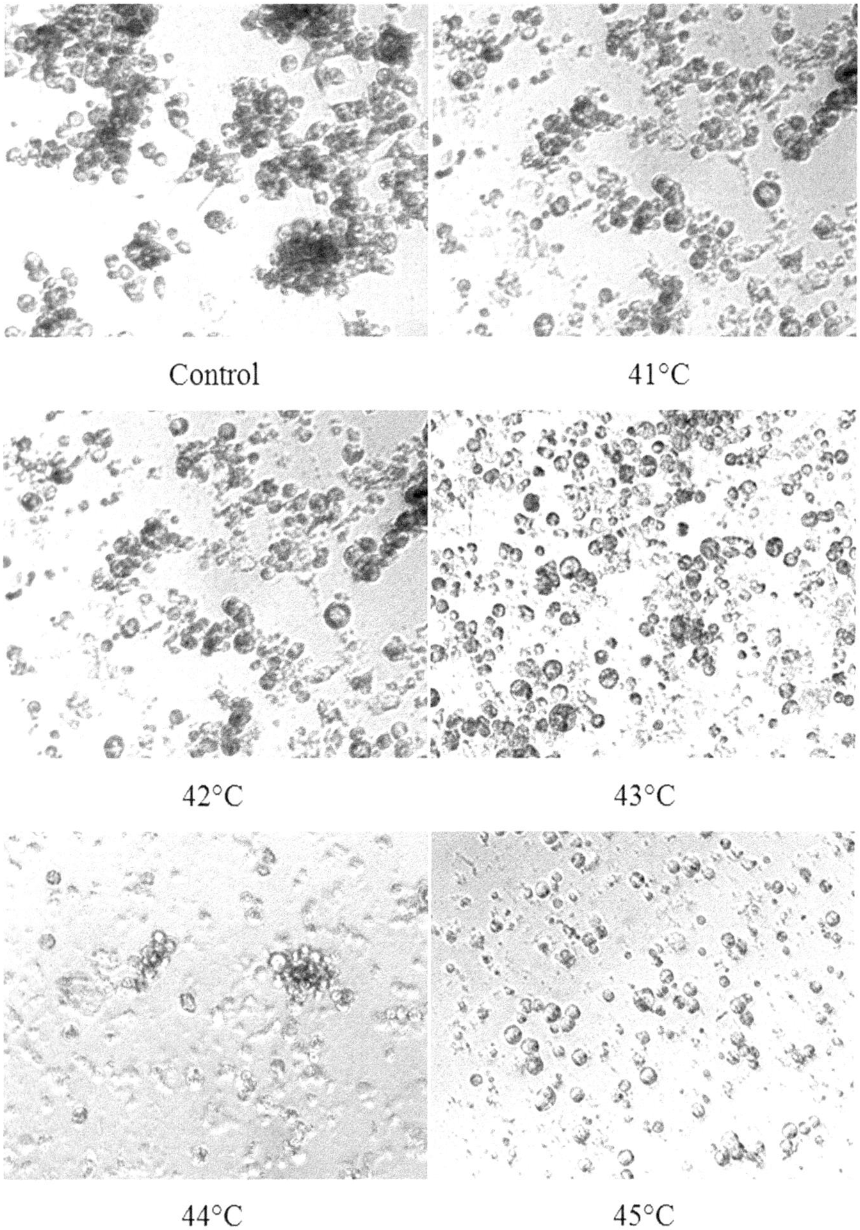

Fig. 5.2 Colon cells on day 2 after heating

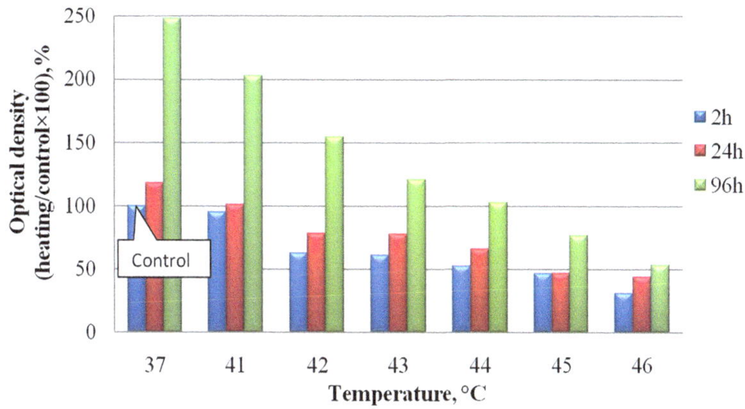

Fig. 5.3 MTT Assay data (Optical density). 2 h, 24 h and 96 h after heating (41–46 °C) Ehrlich cells for 2 h in comparison with control

Thus, high-temperature exposure significantly inhibits proliferate functions of tumor cells only at the temperatures not lower than 44 °C. Temperature regimnes recommended for clinical practice (41–43 °C) have no significant impact on tumor cell viability. Non-transformed (embryonic) cells (CVC, LEC, VERO) are less sensitive to hyperthermia than tumor cells.

5.2 Impact of Hyperthermia on Proliferative Activity of Tumor Cells *In Vivo*

Suspension of Ehrlich tumor cells in the cultural medium RPMI-1640 was heated at 41–50 °C (control cells – at 37 °C) for 2 h. The number of living cells was calculated after trypan blue staining. The cells were concentrated by centrifugation. The cells were inoculated into mice subcutaneously at the dose of 500,000 cells/mouse or intraperitoneally – 1 500,000 cells/mouse. Physiological sodium chloride solution was administered into control animals.

The animals bearing inoculated Ehrlich tumor cells, that were heated at 42 °C and 43 °C prior to inoculation, had a significantly decreased volume of malignant lesions as compared with the control animals and animals after injection of cells treated at 41 °C. Similar data were received in the study of the dynamics of malignant ascites accumulation in mice with intraperitoneally inoculated Ehrlich tumor cells. However, the lack of tumor growth or accumulation of malignant ascites was registered only in those animals that were inoculated with tumor cells warmed at 44 °C prior to inoculation. Incubation of tumor cells in hyperthermic regimen of 41 °C had no any impact on tumor growth (Figs. 5.4, 5.5, and 5.6).

The results demonstrate minimal inhibitory effect of hyperthermic factor on tumor growth at 41 °C and a moderate effect at 42 °C.

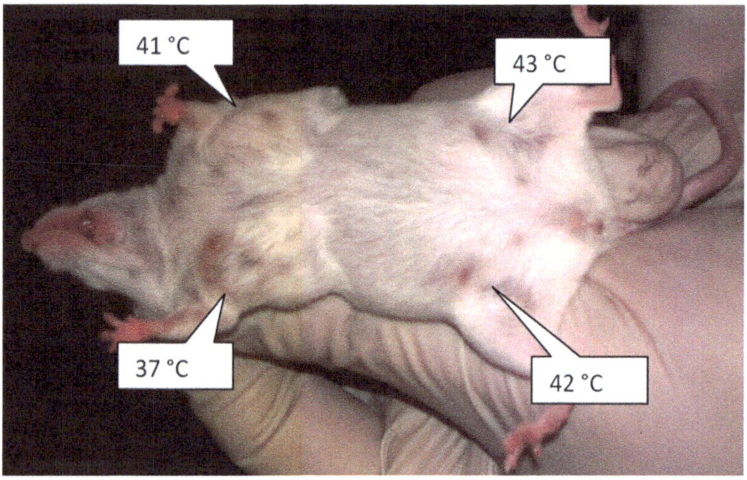

Fig. 5.4 Tumor nodes formation after subcutaneus injection of Ehrlich cells heated at 37 (control), 41, 42 and 43 °C for 2 h. The photo was made 18 days after the injection

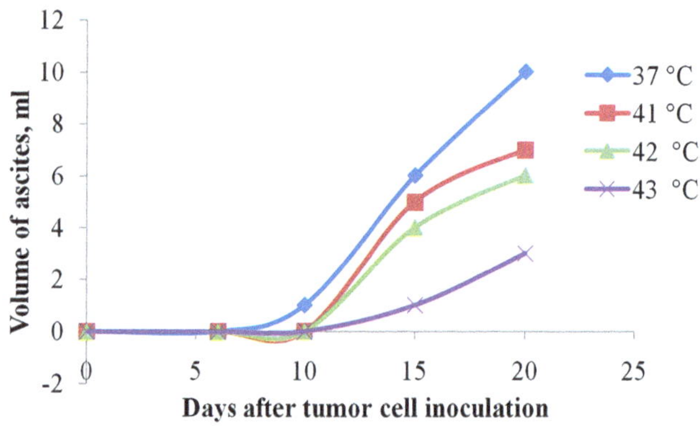

Fig. 5.5 Increase of ascites volume after Ehrlich tumor cells heating prior to intraperitoneal injection

5.3 Effects of Anticancer Drugs and Their Combination with Hyperthermia on the Viability of Tumor Cells *In Vitro*

We suggested using the solutions of anticancer drugs "Cisplatin-Ebewe" or "Mitomycin C Kiowa" and their combination (1:1) heated at high temperature in order to avoid heating the patient's cells up to super high temperatures and/or to reduce anticancer drug doses without any decrease of their effectiveness. The data in Fig. 5.7 show that the cell viability significantly decreases (below 30%) after

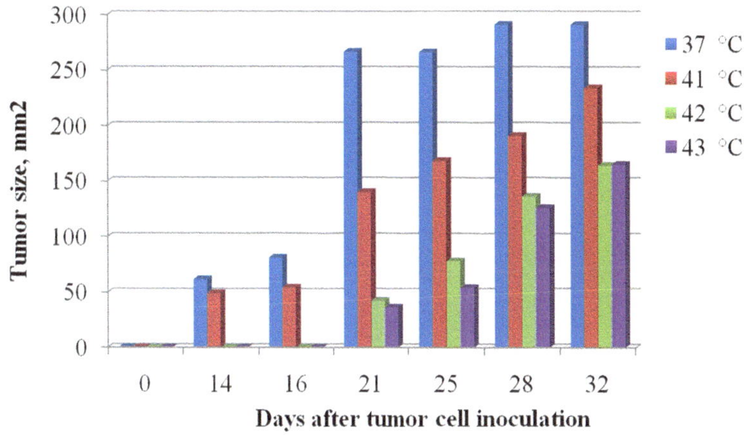

Fig. 5.6 Size of Ehrlich tumor in relation to the cell incubation temperature

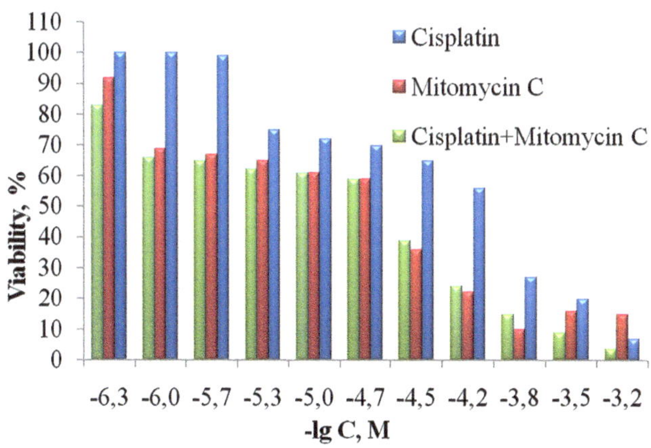

Fig. 5.7 Viability of the Colon cells after incubation for 2 h with Cisplatin or/and Mitomycin C

exposure to the tested anticancer drugs at the concentration of 1.5×10^{-4} M and higher. The difference between the effects of the two drugs and their combination is insignificant.

Combination of anticancer drugs with hyperthermia results in a more pronounced cytotoxic effect as compared with anticancer drugs alone. In particular, we observed inhibition of cell viability by over 50% during their incubation with the drugs at a concentration corresponding to IC50 and being heated at ≥43 °C for 2 h (Fig. 5.8).

Therefore, enhancement of cytostatic effect of anticancer drugs may be achieved only if the temperature of the drug solution reaches 43 °C or higher.

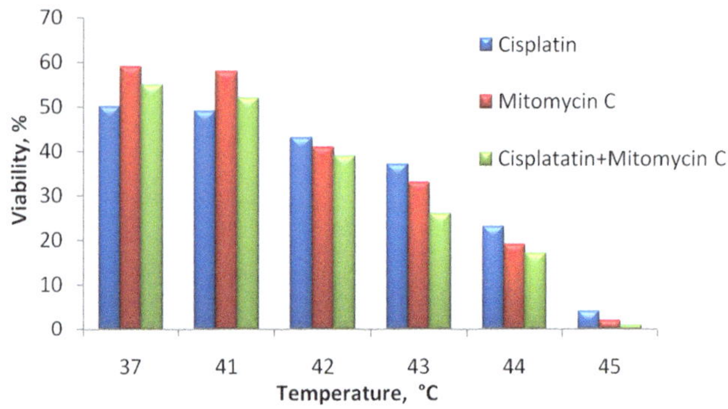

Fig. 5.8 Viability of Colon cells in the presence of Cisplatin ($IC_{50} = 7.5 \times 10^{-5}$ M) and Mitomycin ($IC_{50} = 1.7 \times 10^{-5}$ M) and their combination in the culture medium in the conditions of high temperature exposure (incubation time 2 h). Control - the intact cells incubated at 37 °C

5.4 Effect of Hyperthermia on the Effectors of Antitumor Immunity

Literature reports have shown that the increase of the temperature in the range of 39–40 °C enhances killer function of the effectors of antitumor immunity and the exposure period and tumor microenvironment play an important role [6, 7]. On the one hand, natural killer cells increased their anticancer cytotoxic function after treatment during 2 h in vivo at the temperature of up to 39.5 °C. On the other hand, the cells treated at the temperatures that exceed physiological variability (over 42 °C) for 1 h lead to the decrease of lymphocyte killer activity, which is considered as inhibition of antitumor immunity [8, 9].

Some reports presented the results showing that tumor cells exposed to hyperthermia alone or in combination with anticancer drugs became more sensitive to the action of the activated effectors of antitumor immunity due to the expression of heat shock proteins [10, 11].

To support these data we set a number of experiments where lymphokine-activated killers (LAK) were used as immune effectors. LAK cytotoxic activity was tested in the assays against Colon cells (human colorectal cancer). The results demonstrated that LAK (lymphocytes of healthy volunteers, activated by IL-2) can lyse about 40% of intact tumor cells. However, their cytotoxic effect increased up to 81–89% when tumor cells were preliminary incubated in the medium heated up to 42 °C for 2 h in the presence of Cisplatin and/or Mitomycin C (Fig. 5.9).

This study demonstrated that tumor cell sensitivity increases after cell exposure to heated to 39 °C anticancer drugs.

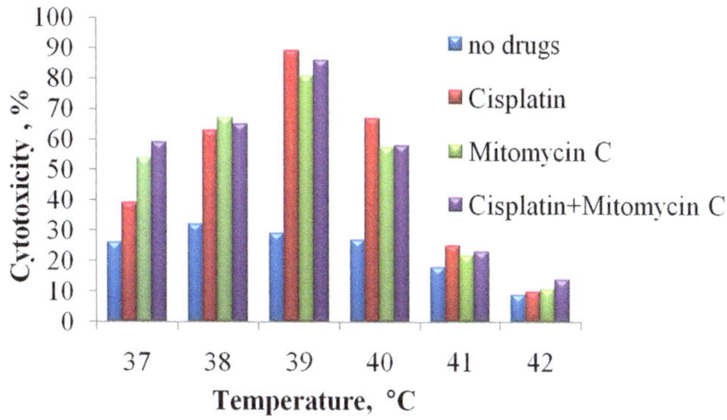

Fig. 5.9 Cytotoxicity of LAK against Colon cells after 2 h of incubation with anticancer drugs in combination with hyperthermia

5.5 Conclusion

The analysis of hyperthermia effect on physiological activity of tumor and non-transformed cells *in vitro* and *in vivo* demonstrated that the damaging and killing effect on tumor cells increases with increasing temperature and time exposure. Like our previous studies, this study showed that the most effective regimen was the following: temperature – 44 °C or higher, exposure time – 2 h or longer. However such regimen of cell treating procedure is difficult to introduce in the patient's organism in clinical settings due to limited tolerance of healthy tissues [12]. Nevertheless, the obtained data clearly demonstrate that the temperature regimes currently recommended for clinical practice (41–43 °C) have no significant impact on viability of tumor cells. Experiments on mice with inoculated Ehrlich tumor cells showed that inhibition of tumor growth was observed only in case if tumor cells were heated at 44 °C prior to injection.

Therefore, when using hyperthermia alone, it is not possible to achieve a significant inhibitory effect on tumor cells. At the same time, incubation of Colon tumor cells in medium with anticancer drugs (Cisplatin or/and Mitomycin C) heated to 42–45 °C provided effective decrease of cell viability to 1–43%. The study also demonstrated that treatment of the cells by anticancer drugs at the temperature of 43 °C increased tumor cell sensitivity to activated lymphocytes. The data proved it reasonable to combine intraperitoneal adoptive immunotherapy with autologous activated lymphocytes – LAK cells, that showed high clinical effectiveness for treatment of malignant effusions in mono-regimen [13, 14].

References

1. Elias D, Raynard B, Boige V, Laplanche A, Estphan G, Malka D, Pocard M (2005) Impact of the extent and duration of cytoreductive surgery on postoperative hematological toxicity after intraperitoneal chemohyperthermia for peritoneal carcinomatosis. J Surg Oncol 90:220–225
2. Baronzio G (2012) Hyperthermia and intracavitary chemotherapy in prevention and treatment of malignant effusions. In: Kiselevsky MV (ed) Malignant effusions: pleuritis, ascites, pericardites. Springer, Dordrecht/New York, pp 123–150
3. Glehen O, Cotte E, Brigand C, Arvieux C, Sayag-Beaujard AC, FN G (2006) Therapeutic innovations in the management of peritoneal carcinomatosis from digestive origin: Cytoreductive surgery and intraperitoneal chemotherapy. Rev Med Int 27:382–391
4. Smeenk RM, Verwaal VJ, Zoetmulder FA (2006) Toxicity and mortality of cytoreduction and intraoperative hyperthermic intraperitoneal chemotherapy in pseudomyxoma peritonei – A report of 103 procedures. Eur J Surg Oncol 32:186–190
5. Bevanda M, Orsolic N, Basic I, Vukojevic K, Benkovic V, Horvat Knezevic A, Lisicic D, Dikic D et al (2009) Prevention of peritoneal carcinomatosis in mice with combination hyperthermal intraperitoneal chemotherapy and IL-2. Int J Hyperth 25(2):132–140
6. Fuggetta MP, Alvino E, Tricarico M, D'Atri S, Pepponi R, Prete SP, Bonmassar E (2000) Adjuvant chemotherapy in gastric cancer: 5-year results of a randomised study by the Italian Trials in Medical Oncology (ITMO) Group. Anticancer Res 20(3A):1667–1672
7. Takeda T, Fukunaga K, Miyazawa K, Takahashi T, Takeda H, Takeda Y, Tanigawa K, Morisaki T, Yamamoto I, Hasegawa T (2008) Immuno-cellular therapy-basic and clinical study. Int J Hyperthermia. Gan To Kagaku Ryoho 35(12):2244–2246
8. Bajetta E, Buzzoni R, Mariani L, Beretta E, Bozzetti F, Bordogna G, Aitini E, Fava S, Schieppati G, Pinotti G, Visini M, Ianniello G, Di BM (2002) In vitro effect of hyperthermia on natural cell-mediated cytotoxicity. Ann Oncol 13(2):299–307
9. Dayanc BE, Beachy SH, Ostberg JR, Repasky EA (2008) Dissecting the role of hyperthermia in natural killer cell mediated anti-tumor responses. Int J Hyperth 24(1):41–45
10. Milani V, Noessner E (2006) Effects of thermal stress on tumor antigenicity and recognition by immune effector cells. Cancer Immunol Immunother 55(3):312–319
11. Moseley P (2000, July 25) Stress proteins and the immune response. Immunopharmacology 48(3):299–302
12. Anisimova NY, Kiselevskiy MV, Abdullaev AG, Malakhova NV, Sitdikova SM, Polotskiy BE, Davydov MM (2016) Effect of hyperthermia on the viability and proliferative activity of tumor cells. Russian Oncol J 21(5):250–252
13. Shubina IZ, Bliumenberg AG, Volkov SM, Demidov LV, Kiselevsky MV (2007) Adoptive immunotherapy of malignancies. Vestn Ross Akad Med Nauk 11:9–15
14. Shubina IZ, Titov KS, Mikhailova IN, Kiselevsky MV (2014) Looking into the future of immunotherapy or how to find Cinderella? Int J Cancer Prev 6(3–4):413–424

Chapter 6
Immunotherapy of Malignant Peritoneal Mesothelioma and Pseudomyxoma Peritonei

Irina Zh. Zhubina, Irina O. Chikileva, and Mikhail V. Kiselevskiy

Abstract Immunotherapy of malignant peritoneal mesothelioma and pseudomixoma peritonei is a promising method and is actively developed to treat patients with these malignancies. The approach includes methods of adoptive cellular immunotherapy with local infusions of autologic activated or genetically modified lymphocytes and target drugs based on monoclonal antibodies, including immune checkpoint inhibitors.

Keywords Immunotherapy · LAK-cells · CAR-T-cells · Immune checkpoint inhibitors

Current approaches to treatment of malignant mesothelioma (MM) include systemic chemotherapy and multimodal therapy: surgical resection combined with chemotherapy and/or radiotherapy; photodynamic therapy and hyperthermic pleural perfusion with subsequent resection [1]. MM is almost insensitive to radiation, since total efficiency of radiotherapy is limited by the dose causing marked adverse effects. That is why radiotherapy is commonly used for palliative purposes in combination with surgical intervention [2, 3]. Patients with peritoneal MM die within 2 years from the diagnosis since this MM type is refractory to all available radio- and chemotherapy methods. At present, there are no any efficient clinical protocols for treatment of this disease. Prognosis for MM patients remains unfavorable with median overall survival (OS) ranging from 13 to 19 months [4].

Over the last decades different schemes have been developed to enhance efficacy of MM treatment including modern target drugs and different methods of adoptive immunotherapy. However, almost all variants of experimental treatment methods as 2nd or subsequent therapy lines failed to show significant anti-cancer efficiency [5].

I. Z. Zhubina (✉) · I. O. Chikileva · M. V. Kiselevskiy
Laboratory of Cell Immunity, N.N. Blokhin National Medical Research Center, Moscow, Russia

© Springer Nature Switzerland AG 2019

M. V. Kiselevskiy et al. (eds.), *Malignant Mesothelioma and Pseudomyxoma*,
https://doi.org/10.1007/978-3-319-99510-6_6

6.1 Adoptive Immunotherapy

MM is considered an immunogenic cancer type as there are cases of spontaneous regression; tumors are infiltrated by immune cells and MM cells are destroyed as a result of immune-cell-mediated killing. Therefore, elucidation of immune system role in MM pathogenesis and development of methods to enhance antitumor immune response or overcome immune suppression might promote elaboration of MM immunotherapy strategies. So far, more than 40 clinical trials applying activated lymphocytes and more than 30 using dendritic-cell (DC)-based vaccines have been started to treat malignant melanoma. However, there are few clinical studies of phase I/II applying activated lymphocytes or DC-vaccines for MM treatment. Although, it is important, autologic cytotoxic T cells against mesothelioma cells may be generated in experimental conditions [6].

Scientific and clinical studies of the 90s proved efficiency of adoptive immunotherapy by recombinant IL-2 (rIL-2) and lymphokine-activated killer cells (LAK) intracavitary infusions in cancer patients with pleuritis and/or ascites (Fig. 6.1). Such adoptive immunotherapy technique allowed creating an effective concentration of cytokines and LAK cells at the tumor site, thus causing lysis of tumor cells without damage of normal tissues. A Phase I-II clinical study of intrapleural IL-2 infusion involving 23 patients with mesothelioma showed response in 19% of the patients along with good tolerance of the treatment [7]. The results of a pilot study of intracavitary infusion of autologic LAK-cells generated from effusion

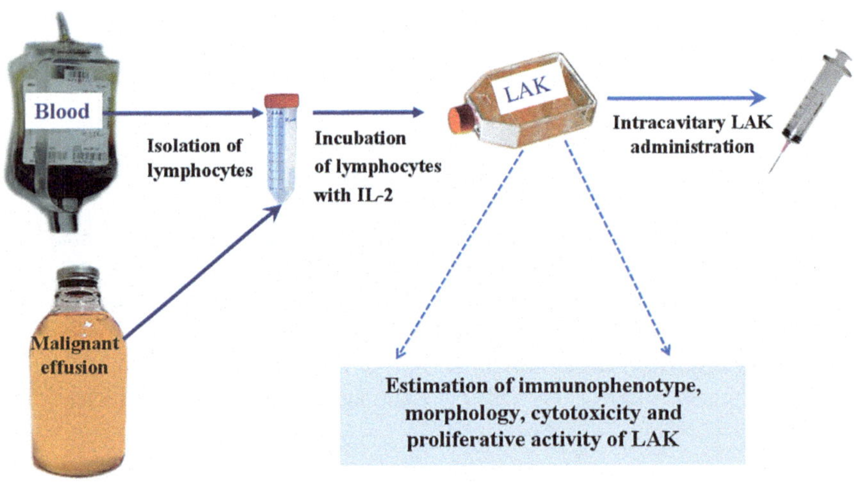

Fig. 6.1 Generation of LAK-cells from peripheral blood and malignant effusion of patients with malignant mesothelioma [8]

- Isolation of lymphocytes; ex vivo incubation of lymphocytes with IL-2
- Analyzing immunophenotype, morphological characteristics, cytotoxic and prolipherative activity of LAK-cells;
- Intracavitary infusion of LAK-cells

lymphocytes combined with IL-2 showed regression of malignant effusion in 5 patients with mesothelioma. Decrease of malignant effusion accumulation was associated with tumor cell degradation. These limited clinical studies presented good promise of IL-2/LAK immunotherapy, since such approach adds to MM treatment methods. The advantages include appropriate tolerance and efficiency of intracavitary infusion [8] (Fig. 6.2). Although the method does not induce complete tumor regression, it allows effective arrest of malignant effusion accumulation. A great promise of the method is also endowed by possible infusion of systemic chemo- and/or radiotherapy after malignant effusion cessation.

Tumor-infiltrating lymphocytes (TILs) were used for MM treatment as well. A phase I/II clinical trial showed efficacy of TIL infusion combined with low-dose interleukin-2 (IL-2). Adoptive immunotherapy followed a preparatory regimen of non-myeloablative lymphodepletion using cyclophosphamide and fludarabine in patients with malignant pleural mesothelioma (MPM). Cyclophosphamide (60 mg/kg/day × 2 days), and fludarabine (25 mg/m^2/day × 5 days) were administrated intravenously (i.v.). Autologous TILs 10×10^{10} were administrated i.v. and low-dose IL-2 was injected subcutaneously (125,000 IU/kg per day) for 2 weeks (with a 2-day interval between each week) [9]. Although the results of the adoptive TIL/

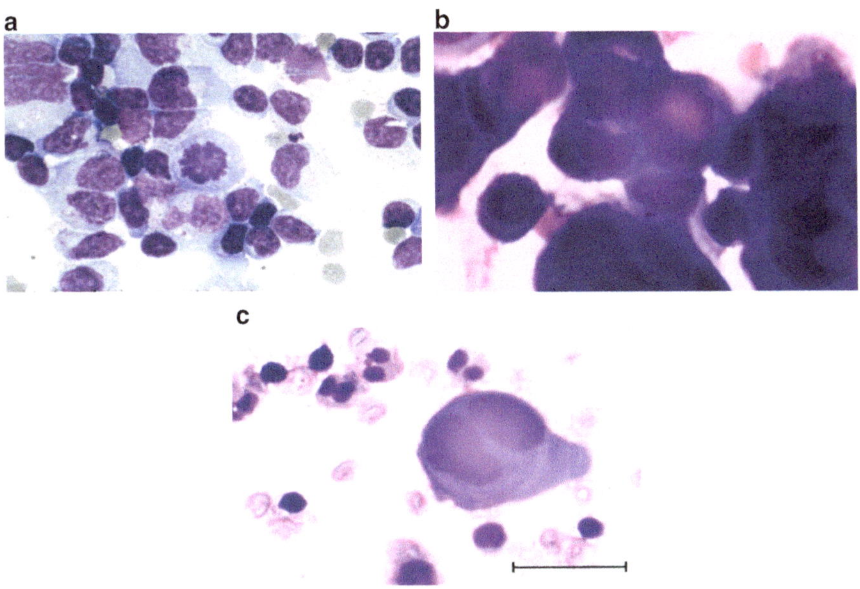

Fig. 6.2 Cytological image of malignant effusion of a patient with malignant mesothelioma before intracavitary immunotherapy with LAK-cells (**a**), at the beginning of IL-2-LAK therapy (**b**) and at the end of IL-2-LAK therapy (**c**) [8]. H&E Staining, original magnification ×900
Initally malignant effusion includes mesothelioma cells and single lymphocytes. LAK-cells are represented by activated and proliferating lymphocytes of immunoblast-like cells and prolymphocytes. At the end of the immunotherapy course the residual effusion presents single mesothelioma cells in degradation.

IL-2-therapy have not been published yet, it is reasonable to assume good persepc-tive of this method for MM treatment. A clinical study combining DC and cytokine-induced killer (CIK) cells in MM adoptive immunotherapy will be accomplished soon. Cells were re-infused to the patients 3 times intravenously. Patients will receive at least 2 cycles of DC-CIK (Table 6.1).

6.2 Dendritic Cell-Based Cancer Therapeutic Vaccines

Dendritic cells (DCs) are professional antigen-presenting cells (APCs) that drive T cell-mediated immune responses. Vaccination with DCs pulsed with tumor lysates increases therapeutic antitumor immune responses both in vitro and in vivo Several studies of dindritic cell vaccines (DC-vaccines) as therapeutic agent were perfomed for MM treatment. Most of them used lysates of autologous tumors as a source of tumor antigen because mesothelioma-specific tumor-associated antigens (TAAs) have not been identified, yet. However, this approach excludes patients with unavailable tumor material. One of the studies involved 6 MM patients [10]. Clinical efficiency was evaluated according to the modified Response Evaluation Criteria in Solid Tumors (modified RECIST) and included 3 patients with partial responses and one with stable disease after DC-immunotherapy. It should be emphasized, however, that even in patients with a registered clinical effect the survival period between diagnosis and death did not exceed a year. Another pilot study of a DC-vaccine, using the lysate of an allogeneic tumor, showed partial response in 2 patients from 9; 7 patients had stable disease, median progression free survival was 8.3 months [11]. DC-vaccine studies utilizing synthetic peptides as antigens, WT-1 in particular, will continue, the method does not require tumor material and may be standardized. However, in the authors' opinion, this approach is limited by antitumor response to only one peptide. As most of tumors are highly heterogenic and consist of different tumor clones, expressing divergent TAAs, elimination of a tumor clone does not exclude proliferation of the others [12]. Different strategies are currently being studied for MM treatment. DC-based therapy is still regarded as a promising way of MM treatment.

6.3 Target Drugs

A few target drugs were evaluated in mesothelioma treatment. As angiogenesis is a key event in carcinogenesis its inhibitors were considered a good potential for MM treatment [13]. Clinical trials of angiogenesis inhibitors with different mechanisms of action were performed to evaluate their efficacy. However, the results were rather modest with response rates of 0–23% and overall survival of 5.9–12.4 months. Thus, Thalidomide, the most extensively studied drug, did not provide significant improvement as the first line of MM therapy [14]. Anti-VEGF antibody Bevacizumab

Table 6.1 Clinical trials of adoptive immunotherapy for treatment of malignant mesothelioma

Agent	Phase	Clinical trials	Comments	Clinical Trials. gov identifier (NCT number)
TILs	I/II	Study Evaluating the Infusion of Tumor-Infiltrating Lymphocytes (TILs) and Low-Dose Interleukin-2 (IL-2) Therapy Following a Preparative Regimen of Non-myeloablative Lymphodepletion Using Cyclophosphamide and Fludarabine in Patients With Malignant Pleural Mesothelioma	Prior to the cell infusion, patients will receive two drugs cyclophosphamide and fludarabine. After cell infusion, patients will receive low-dose interleukin-2	NCT02414945
DC-CIK	I/II	Combination of Immunotherapy and Hyperthermia in Advanced Malignant Mesothelioma	Patients will receive pembrolizumab 100 mg every 3 weeks until disease progression, unacceptable toxicity or patient refusal. Patients will receive at least 2 cycles of DC-CIK Immunotherapy along with 4 dosage of anti-PD-1 antibody treatment Hyperthermia for 40 min, with maximum temperature settled on 42 °C ± 0.5 °C as upper limit, twice a week since the 1st week of pembrolizumab for a total of 10 times.	NCT03393858
DC-vaccine	I	Dendritic Cell-based Immunotherapy Combined With Low-dose Cyclophosphamide in Patients With Malignant Mesothelioma (PMR-MM-002)	4 cycles of chemotherapy. DCs are cultured in vitro and pulsed with tumor lysate. 3 doses of autologous DC-vaccine (MesoCancerVac) are re-injected every 2 weeks.	NCT01241682
DC-vaccine	I	Dendritic Cell-based Immunotherapy in Mesothelioma	4 courses of chemotherapy (Alimta/cisplatin). 3 doses of properly pulsed autologous dendritic cells are then re-injected every 2 weeks.	NCT00280982

(continued)

Table 6.1 (continued)

Agent	Phase	Clinical trials	Comments	Clinical Trials. gov identifier (NCT number)
DC-vaccine	I	Autologous Dendritic Cell Vaccination in Mesothelioma (MESODEC)	Four 3-weekly cycles of platinum/pemetrexed four intradermal vaccinations with 8–10 × 10^6 autologous WT1 mRNA-loaded DCs	NCT02649829
DC-vaccine	I	αDC1 Vaccine + Chemokine Modulatory Regimen (CKM) as Adjuvant Treatment of Peritoneal Surface Malignancies	Autologous alpha-type-1 polarized dendritic cell (alpha-DC1) vaccines (patients' autologous alpha-DC1s loaded with autologous tumor material), combined with a systemic chemokine modulation regimen [CKM; intravenous rintatolimod (TLR3 ligand, a derivative of Poly-I:C) + intravenous interferon-alfa + oral celecoxib] as adjuvant therapy, after cytoreductive surgery (CRS) and hyperthermic intraperitoneal chemotherapy (HIPEC),	NCT02151448
DC-vaccine	I/II	Dendritic Cell Vaccination for Patients With Solid Tumors	4 biweekly intradermal vaccinations with autologous RNA- modified DCs-engineered to express the WT1 protein	NCT01291420
anti-fibroblast activation protein CAR-T cells	I	Re-directed T Cells for the Treatment (FAP)-Positive Malignant Pleural Mesothelioma	single dose of 1 × 10^6 adoptively transferred FAP-specific re-directed T cells given directly in the pleural effusion	NCT01722149
anti-mesothelin CAR-T cells	I	CAR T Cells in Mesothelin Expressing Cancers	Intravenously or intrapleurally administered lentiviral transduced huCART-meso cells with or without lymphodepletion	NCT03054298

(continued)

Table 6.1 (continued)

Agent	Phase	Clinical trials	Comments	Clinical Trials. gov identifier (NCT number)
anti-mesothelin CAR-T cells	I	Treatment of Relapsed and/or Chemotherapy Refractory Advanced Malignancies by CART-meso	Anti-meso-CAR retroviral vector-transduced autologous T cells. 3 doses in the absence of disease progression or unacceptable toxicity.	NCT02580747
anti-mesothelin -CAR T cells	I	Autologous Redirected RNA Meso-CAR T Cells	1. One dose of 1×10^8 cells followed by one dose of 1×10^9 autologous transfected anti-mesothelin CAR T.	NCT01355965
			2. Three doses of 1×10^8 cells followed by three doses of 1×10^9 T cells	
anti-mesothelin -CAR T cells	I	Malignant Pleural Disease Treated With Autologous T Cells Genetically Engineered to Target the Cancer-Cell Surface Antigen Mesothelin	Mesothelin-targeted T cells administered intrapleurally as a single infusion. A maximum dose of 3×10^6 mesothelin-targeted T cells/kg	NCT02414269

in combination with chemotherapy in European clinical studies demonstrated ambiguous results [15]. MM expresses VEGFR, PDGFR, as well as cKIT. That is why Sorafenib, a potent inhibitor of the RAS/RAF/MEK pathway, which also targets VEGFR and cKIT was studied in MM therapy. 51 patients were enrolled in the study. Three patients had a partial response (6%), and 27 had stable disease. Median progression-free survival and median overall survival were 3.6 months and 9.7 months, respectively [16].

Transforming growth factor β (TGF-β) is a pleiotropic cytokine and a potential growth inhibitor in normal conditions. TGF-β promotes remodelling microenvironment for tumor growth support, facilitates metastasis and suppresses antitumor immune reactions. Elevated plasma TGF-β levels correlate with advanced cancer grade, metastases and poor survival. GC1008 (Fresolimumab), humanized monoclonal antibody neutralizes all three human TGF-β isoforms. The trial was designed as a 40 open-label, phase II trial for patients with relapsed MPM(NCT01112293). Stable disease was noted after 4 courses in 3 of the 13 patients (23%). Nevertheless, despite the lack of radiographic response and short progression-free survival time, the 12 month median overall survival was reported, with one patient still alive more than 25 months after treatment [17].

6.4 Immune Checkpoint Inhibitors

T cells infiltrating tumors are usually anergic as they up-regulate so-called immune checkpoints – receptors capable of inhibiting immune response. The most widely known immune checkpoints are cytotoxic lymphocyte antigen-4 (CTLA-4) and programmed cell death 1 (PD-1) receptors [18]. Tumors often express PD-1 ligand (PD-L1), which suppresses tumor lysis through ligation of PD-1 on immune CTLs. As many other tumors, MM possesses high levels of immunosuppressive PD-L1 [19]. The idea to block immune checkpoints or their ligands to enhance antitumor immune reactions has been proved effective. Monoclonal antibodies against CTLA-4 (Tremelimumab, Ipilimumab), PD-1 (Nivolumab, Pembrolizumab) and PD-L1 (Avelumab, MPDL3280A) may elevate antitumor immune response and demonstrate significant clinical efficiency in treatment of melanoma and certain other cancer types.

So far, several clinical studies testing immune checkpoint inhibitors in MM treatment have been completed. In particular, phase II trial of CTLA-4 blocking antibody, Tremelimumab, in the dose of 15 mg/kg, showed its clinical efficacy in 38% of MM patients [20]. More intensive regimen (Tremelimumab 10 mg/kg once every 4 weeks for six doses, then every 12 weeks until disease progression, unacceptable toxic effects, or refusal to continue the treatment) proved to be safe enough. More than 40% of MM patients had disease stabilization with medium response rate of almost 11 months [21]. The same intensive regimen was studied in a randomized phase IIb study (NCT01843374). Other clinical trials of PD-1 inhibitor Pembrolizumab (NCT02399371) and PD-L1-blocker Avelumab (NCT01772004) are still on-going. The recently published results of KEYNOTE-028 study showed good tolerance of Pembrolizumab and clinical improvement in MM patients. Partial response accounted for 28%, while 48% of the patients had disease stabilization. Response rate to this immune checkpoint inhibitor was much higher as compared with the second line chemotherapy [22]. Recently a large clinical study «DETERMINE» (phase IIb trial) has been completed. It included 569 patients with advanced unresectable pleural or peritoneal malignant mesothelioma. 380 of the patients received Tremelimumab and 189 – placebo. At the cutoff date 307 (80%) patients died in the Tremelimumab arm and 154 (81%) of the patients died in the placebo arm. Medians of overall survival did not differ between the groups and comprised 7.7 months for Tremelimumab and 7.3 for the placebo arms. Treatment associated adverse events of grade 3 or worse occurred in 65% of the patients in the Tremelimumab arm and in 4 (8%) of the placebo arm. Thus, Tremelimumab did not significantly improve overall survival compared to placebo in patients with previously treated malignant mesothelioma. Tremelimumab safety profile was equivalent to the known profile of CTLA-4 inhibitors. Currently, there are on-going studies with the aim of showing if combined immunotherapy might be more effective then monotherapy for MM treatment [23]. On the whole, immune checkpoint inhibitors are the agents of the most promising types of new molecules for MM treatment, which is supported by multiple on-going clinical trials of checkpoint inhibitors and their combinations in MM therapy (Table 6.2).

Table 6.2 Clinical trials of Checkpoint inhibitors for the treatment of malignant mesothelioma

Agent	Phase	Clinical trials	Comments	Clinical Trials.gov identifier (NCT number)
Ipilimumab and Nivolumab	II	Ipilimumab and Nivolumab in the Treatment of Malignant Pleural Mesothelioma (INITIATE)	Nivolumab administered at a fixed dose of 240 mg every 2 weeks for a maximum period of 2 years. Nivolumab will be given in combination with ipilimumab on week 1, 7, 13 and 19. Ipilimumab administered at the dose of 1 mg/Kg.	NCT03048474
Nivolumab	II	Nivolumab in Patients With Recurrent Malignant Mesothelioma (NivoMes)	Nivolumab administered 2 times weekly by intravenous infusion in a dose of 3 mg/kg	NCT02497508
Nivolumab Monotherapy or Nivolumab Plus Ipilimumab	II	Nivolumab Monotherapy or Nivolumab Plus Ipilimumab, for Unresectable Malignant Pleural Mesothelioma (MPM) Patients (MAPS2)	*Monotherapy Arm*	NCT02716272
			Nivolumab administered at 3 mg/kg every 2 weeks	
			Combination Arm	
			Nivolumab administered IV over 60 min at 3 mg/kg every 2 weeks, combined with Ipilimumab administered IV over 90 min at 1 mg/Kg every 6 weeks	
Nivolumab	III	Checkpoint Blockade For Inhibition of Relapsed Mesothelioma (CONFIRM)	Nivolumab 240 mg until disease progression, to a maximum of 12 months.	NCT03063450
			Placebo	
			Sterile 0.9% sodium chloride	
IPI-549 is a potent and selective phosphoinositide-3-kinase (PI3Kγ) Inhibitor and Nivolumab		A Dose-Escalation Study to Evaluate the Safety, Tolerability, Pharmacokinetics, and Pharmacodynamics of IPI-549		NCT02637531

(continued)

Table 6.2 (continued)

Agent	Phase	Clinical trials	Comments	Clinical Trials.gov identifier (NCT number)
Ipilimumab Nivolumab	II	Study of Nivolumab Combined With Ipilimumab Versus Pemetrexed and Cisplatin or Carboplatin as First Line Therapy in Unresectable Pleural Mesothelioma Patients (CheckMate743)	Randomized, Open Label Trial of Nivolumab in Combination With Ipilimumab Versus Pemetrexed With Cisplatin or Carboplatin as First Line Therapy in Unresectable Pleural Mesothelioma	NCT02899299
INCAGN01876 combined with nivolumab.	II	Phase 1/2 Study Exploring the Safety, Tolerability, and Efficacy of INCAGN01876 Combined With Immune Therapies in Advanced or Metastatic Malignancies	INCAGN01876 combined with nivolumab.	NCT03126110
INCAGN01876 combined with Ipilimumab			INCAGN01876 combined with ipilimumab. NCAGN01876 combined with Nivolumab and Ipilimumab.	
ABBV-368 (anti–c-Met antibody) nivolumab		A Study of the Safety, Tolerability and Pharmacokinetics of as a Single Agent and Combination in Subjects With Locally Advanced or Metastatic Solid Tumors	ABBV-368 as a monotherapy and in combination with Nivolumab in participants with locally advanced or metastatic solid tumors.	NCT03071757
INCAGN01876 (anti-human glucocorticoid-induced tumor necrosis factor receptor) Nivolumab Ipilimumab	I/II	Phase 1/2 Study Exploring the Safety, Tolerability, and Efficacy of INCAGN01876 Combined With Immune Therapies in Advanced or Metastatic Malignancies	INCAGN01876 combined with Nivolumab. INCAGN01876 combined with Ipilimumab INCAGN01876 combined with Nivolumab and Ipilimumab.	NCT03126110
Pembrolizumab	I	A Pilot Window-Of-Opportunity Study of the Anti-PD-1 Antibody Pembrolizumab in Patients With Resectable Malignant Pleural Mesothelioma	Three courses of Pembrolizumab will be administered (200 mg iv every 21 days)	NCT02707666
Pembrolizumab	I	Adjuvant Pembrolizumab After Radiation Therapy for Lung-Intact Malignant Pleural Mesothelioma	Pembrolizumab after radiation therapy (with or without surgery and/or chemotherapy)	NCT02959463

Pembrolizumab	II	Pembrolizumab in Patients With Advanced Malignant Pleural Mesothelioma	1. Pemetrexed 500 mg/m2 IV Day 1 every 21 days for 6 cycles Cisplatin 75 mg/m2 IV Day 1 every 21 days for 6 cycles	NCT02784171
			2. Pembrolizumab 200 mg* IV Day 1 over 30 min every 21 days for a total of 2 years Pemetrexed 500 mg/m2 IV Day 1 every 21 days for 6 cycles Cisplatin 75 mg/m2 IV Day 1 every 21 days for 6 cycles	
			3. Pembrolizumab 200 mg* IV 30 min Day 1 every 21 days for a total of 2 years	
Pembrolizumab with or without Anetumab (mesothelin-targeting antibody)	I/II	Phase 1 Safety Run-In and Phase 2 Randomized Clinical Trial of Anetumab Ravtansine and MK-3475 (Pembrolizumab) Compared to MK-3475 (Pembrolizumab) Alone for Mesothelin-Positive Malignant Pleural Mesothelioma	1. Patients receive pembrolizumab IV over 30 min on day 1. Courses repeat every 21 days for up to 2 years in the absence of disease progression or unacceptable toxicity. Upon radiologic documentation of disease progression, patients may cross over to Group II.	NCT03126630
			2. Patients receive anetumab ravtansine IV over 1 h and pembrolizumab IV over 30 min on day 1. Courses repeat every 21 days for up to 2 years in the absence of disease progression or unacceptable toxicity.	
Pembrolizumab	III	Pembrolizumab Immunotherapy Versus Standard Chemotherapy for Advanced pre-treated Malignant Pleural Mesothelioma (PROMISE-meso)	Pembrolizumab is administrated at 200 mg fixed dose i.v. on day 1 of every 3 week cycle for a maximum or 2 years (expected maximum of 36 doses), or until progression of disease	NCT02991482

(continued)

Table 6.2 (continued)

Agent	Phase	Clinical trials	Comments	Clinical Trials.gov identifier (NCT number)
Pembrolizumab CRS-207 (live-attenuated, double-deleted Listeria monocytogenes engineered to express the tumor-associated antigen mesothelin)	II	Evaluation of CRS-207 With Pembrolizumab in Previously Treated MPM	CRS-207 and pembrolizumab will be administered in 3-week cycles.	NCT03175172
Pembrolizumab	II	Pembrolizumab in Treating Patients With Malignant Mesothelioma	Pembrolizumab IV over 30 min on day 1. Treatment repeats every 21 days for up to 24 months in the absence of disease progression or unacceptable toxicity	NCT02399371
Pembrolizumab Defactinib (small-molecule focal adhesion kinase (FAK) inhibitor with potential antiangiogenic and antineoplastic activities.)		Study of FAK (Defactinib) and PD-1 (Pembrolizumab) Inhibition in Advanced Solid Malignancies (FAK-PD1)	200 mg (iv) pembrolizumab every 3 weeks; plus 200 mg/400 mg (oral) defactinib twice daily	NCT02758587
Pembrolizumab DC-CIK immunotherapy hyperthermia		Combination of Immunotherapy and Hyperthermia in Advanced Malignant Mesothelioma	anti-PD-1 monoclonal antibody plus autologous dendritic cells-cytokine induced killer cell (DC-CIK) immunotherapy combined with hyperthermia	NCT03393858
CDX-1401 (A fusion protein consisting of a fully human monoclonal antibody directed against the endocytic dendritic cell receptor, DEC-205, linked to the TAA NY-ESO-1, Poly-ICL (a ligand for toll like receptor-3), and Pembrolizumab	I/II	A Trial of CDX-1401 in Combination With Poly-ICLC and Pembrolizumab, in Previously Treated Advanced Solid Tumor Patients	combination of three drugs	NCT02661100

Tremelimumab Anti-PD-L1 (durvalumab)	II	A Study of Tremelimumab Combined With the Anti-PD-L1 MEDI4736 Antibody in Malignant Mesothelioma (NIBIT-MESO-1)	tremelimumab 1 mg/kg i.v over 60 min plus MEDI 4736 20 mg/kg i.v every 3 weeks for 4 doses, then MEDI4736 20 mg/kg IV every 4 weeks for additional 9 doses.	NCT02588131
MEDI4736 (durvalumab) Tremelimumab	II	MEDI4736 or MEDI4736 + Tremelimumab in Surgically Resectable Malignant Pleural Mesothelioma	MEDI4736 (15 mg/kg intravenously, once), 1–6 weeks prior to surgical resection.	NCT02592551
			MEDI4736 (1500 mg intravenously, once) + tremelimumab (75 mg intravenously, once), 1–6 weeks prior to surgical resection.	
CK-301 (fully human monoclonal antibody of IgG1 subtype that directly binds to PD-L1)	I	Phase 1 Study of CK-301 as a Single Agent in Subjects With Advanced Cancers	CK-301 administered in periods of 28 day cycles.	NCT03212404
Arginase Inhibitor INCB001158		Arginase Inhibitor INCB001158 as a Single Agent and in Combination With Immune Checkpoint Therapy in Patients With Advanced/Metastatic Solid Tumors	INCB001158 as a single agent and in combination with immune checkpoint inhibitor	NCT02903914
Pembrolizumab				
Pembrolizumab	II	Study of Pembrolizumab (MK-3475) in Participants With Advanced Solid Tumors (MK-3475-158/KEYNOTE-158)	Pembrolizumab 200 mg intravenously every 3 weeks for up to 35 administrations (approximately 2 years of treatment)	NCT02628067
LAG525 (antibody targets the immune checkpoint LAG-3)		Safety and Efficacy of LAG525 Single Agent and in Combination With PDR001 in Patients With Advanced Malignancies.	Single agent treatment arm with LAG525.	NCT02460224
PDR001 (anti-PD-1)			Combination treatment arm with LAG525 and PDR001	

6.5 Mesothelin and Other MM-Associated Targets for MM Immunotherapy

Altogether with encouraging trials of immune checkpoint inhibitors, promising preclinical studies lead to clinical phase I trials of substances targeting mesothelin.

Mesothelin has low expression rate in most normal tissues, but it is more expressed in many solid tumors, including MM [24]. Biological role of mesothelin overexpression in MM is still unknown. However, data of preclinical studies have demonstrated that it promotes MM tumor cell invasion and matrix metalloprotease secretion [25]. Mesothelin-targeting agents may be subdivided into three categories: (i) anti-cancer antibodies/immunotoxins; (ii) vaccines targeting mesothelin; (iii) mesothelin-targeting recombinant T-cells.

Amatuximab (MORAb-009) is a humanized monoclonal antibody, which showed high activity in preclinical studies in combination with chemotherapy against mesothelin-expressing tumors through blockade of mesothelin interactions [26]. In a phase I clinical trial, Amatuximab demonstrated an appropriate toxicity profile along with moderate activity. 11 patients from 24 (46%) had steady disease stabilization [27]. However, a phase II clinical trial of Amatuximab with Pemetrexed and Cisplatin showed that progression-free survival was not significantly different from historical controls. Altogether, overall survival exceeded historical control and lasted for 14.8 months [28]. A phase III clinical study is planned for detailed evaluation of the results.

Wilms tumor protein 1 (WT1) is a transcription factor, highly expressed in MM and ovarian cancer, which attracted researchers' attention as a potential immunotherapy target. WT1 peptides are immunogenic and induce T-cell reactions against MM-cell lines [29]. There were developed WT1-vaccines, which induced immune response in patients with MM. Phase I clinical studies to evaluate safety of WT-1-based vaccines have been just finished or are still on-going (NCT00398138, NCT01265433, NCT01890980).

Mesothelin-specific CAR-T-cells (CARTmeso) as well as WT1 and FAP-targeting CAR-T-cells will be discussed later.

6.6 Immunotoxins

Recently cytotoxic drugs – immunotoxins based on antibodies against TAAs have been designed for antitumor therapies [30]. In particular, immunotoxin SS1P consists of variable fragment of Amatuximab linked with a bacterial toxin from *Pseudomonas* – exotoxin A [31, 32]. The immunotoxin showed anticancer activity in preclinical studies against mesothelin-expressing tumors. In a phase I clinical trial of SS1P monotherapy lead to moderate antitumor effects [33, 34]. In another phase I clinical trial SS1P was studied together with Pemetrexed and Cisplatin in MM patients; 77% of the patients demonstrated partial response [35]. The authors explained moderate results of the study by formation of SS1P-neutralizing antibodies after the first treatment course. Immune suppression along with Pentostatin and Cyclophosphamide administration to deplete T and B cells effectively prevented production of the neutralizing antibody and allowed more SS1P-therapy courses, which resulted in long-lasting partial effects in 30% of the patients [36]. (NCT01362790).

6.7 CAR-T Cells

CAR-T-cell technology is a promising tool against tumors expressing the defined TAAs. The approach is based on genetically modified T lymphocytes, which express specially engineered receptors (chimeric antigen receptors – CAR) containing variable part of a TAA-specific monoclonal antibody coupled with T-cell-receptor signaling domain [37]. Signaling portions of other immune receptors may be supplementary introduced to enhance CAR activity.

Mesothelin-specific CAR-T cells (CARTmeso) showed significant activity in preclinical studies both *in vitro* and *in vivo*. However, CARTmeso may be inactivated by tumor microenvironment, therefore their combination with immune checkpoint inhibitors are supposed to enhance functional activity of human CAR-T cells. Moreover, a particular way of CARTmeso administration may influence therapy efficiency [38]. Some Phase I studies have started recently (NCT02159716, NCT01583686).

Intrapleural infusion (regional infusion) of CAR-T cells eliminated established pleural tumors more effectively even in a 30-fold lower dose than intravenous CAR-T cells infusion. Additionally, regionally delivered CAR-T cells were able to move effectively from the pleural cavity to both lateral and peritoneal tumor sites, and they induced systemic, long-term, antitumor immune response. Regional infusion of CAR-T cells for locoregionally aggressive solid tumors, such as MPM, provides an opportunity to evaluate regional immune reactions that can be effective alone or in combination with systemic immune therapies [39]. Candidate target antigens currently being studied for CAR-T-cell therapy of MM patients include chondroitin sulfate proteoglycan-4 and fibroblast activation protein; MSLN-targeted, CD28 co-stimulated (M28z).

Similar to mesothelin, CAR-T cells against WT1 have tested for their anti-cancer activity. A phase I clinical study (NCT02408016) is now underway.

A new target for CAR-T cells is fibroblast activation protein (FAP), a protein expressed by cancer-associated fibroblasts of most solid tumors. Moreover, MM tumor cells also express FAP, thus making FAP a more attractive immunotherapy target. The data of preclinical studies demonstrate a highly potential role of FAP for MM treatment [40]. Phase I clinical trial of FAP-CAR T cells is currently recruiting participants. This is a phase I trial for patients with malignant pleural mesothelioma. A fixed single dose of adoptively transferred FAP-specific CD8 positive re-directed T cells will be studied for pleural effusion treatment.

Three patients who were at the time of screening not operable will be treated with re-directed T cells by intrapleural infusion after completion of 3 courses of palliative chemotherapy. The patient number will reach 6 patients in case of one AE grade III/IV or one SAE, and the occurrence of DLT (if considered treatment-related by an independent safety monitoring board). The study will be discontinued if one additional treatment-related DLT occurs.

Patients with pleural effusion will receive intapleural infusion of 1×10^6 re-directed FAP-specific T cells. The study ends 35 days after adoptive T cell transfer. Re-directed FAP-specific T cells will be infused on day 0 (day 14 of the third course of palliative chemotherapy). The study is designed to demonstrate safety of $1\text{x}10^6$ re-directed FAP-specific T cells. The next patient will be enrolled when the previous patient completed day 14 treatment and the safety monitoring board has not declared any DLTs. The palliative chemotherapy is not part of the study protocol, though (NCT01722149).

6.8 Neo-Antigens as Targets

Targeting tumor-specific neo-antigens for purposes of cancer immunotherapy is a promising approach for treatment of chronic lymphocytic leukemia and certain solid tumors [41] and metastatic cholangiocarcinoma [42]. Compared to point mutations, the novel open reading frames (neoORFs) generated by small inserts or deletions could induce highly specific antitumor immunity and could be recognized by T cells [43]. It should be noted that neoORFs may be prioritized because they provide a completely novel protein sequence with no counterpart in any normal cells [44].

A novel frameshift insert somatic mutation in BAP1 was reported in an MM patient's tumor sequencing results [3]. The authors produced a polyclonal antibody against the synthesized 13-mer neo-peptide, which differentially stained during immunohistochemistry (IHC) the neoplastic cells but not the normal tissue. Frameshift mutations in BAP1 are common events in MM, and the neo-antigens could be ideal biomarkers for diagnosis.

6.9 Anti-Cancer Viruses

Viruses may be used as alternative anti-cancer agents. Interest in anti-cancer virotherapy has been constantly increasing over the last decade. Certain intrinsic characteristics of mesothelioma, such as its availability and local dissemination, relative absence of distant metastases, make it a good candidate for virotherapy. Although multiple studies have identified potential efficiency of virotherapy based on a live-attenuated measles virus (MV) for certain cancer types, information on anti-cancer activity of MV-vaccine in mesothelioma is still unavailable [45].

6.10 Immunotherapy of Pseudomyxoma Peritonei

So far, only single cases of immunotherapy strategies for pseudomyxoma peritonei treatment were described. In particular, Blumenberg A & Kiselevskiy M [46] demonstrated partial effect of intraperitoneal adoptive immunotherapy including IL-2 (in the dose of 1 mln IU on days 1, 3, 5, 7 and 9 along with 200 mln allogenic LAK-cells on days 2, 4, 6, 8 and 10).

Only one of 19 clinical protocols for pseudomyxoma treatment implies a possibility of immunotherapy. This is a clinical trial Phase II Nivolumab and Ipilimumab in Treating Patients with Rare Tumors (NCT02834013). In this study patients receive Nivolumab i.v. for 30 min on days 1, 15, and 29 and Ipilimumab i.v. for 60 min on day 1. Courses repeat every 42 days in the absence of disease progression or unacceptable toxicity. The trialis are planned to be accomplished by 2020.

6.11 Conclusion

Immunotherapy is a promising strategy for MM treatment as a monotherapy and in combination with other treatment modalities, which has been demonstrated by a number of studies in different lines of therapy. Obviously, target therapy and immunotherapy strategies should prove their clinical efficacy in pleural mesothelioma and pseudomyxoma treatment in the future.

References

1. Zervos MD, Bizekis C, Pass HI (2008) Malignant mesothelioma 2008. Curr Opin Pulm Med 14(4):303–309
2. Bononi A, Napolitano A, Pass H, Yang H, Carbone M (2015) Latest developments in our understanding of the pathogenesis of mesothelioma and the design of targeted therapies. Expert Rev Respir Med 9(5):633–654. https://doi.org/10.1586/17476348.2015.1081066
3. Lai J, Zhou Z, Tang XJ, Gao ZB, Zhou J, Chen SQ (2016) A tumor-specific neo-antigen caused by a frameshift mutation in BAP1 is a potential personalized biomarker in malignant peritoneal mesothelioma. Int J Mol Sci 17(5):pii: E739. https://doi.org/10.3390/ijms17050739
4. Vogelzang NJ, Rusthoven JJ, Symanowski J et al (2003) Phase III study of pemetrexed in combination with cisplatin versus cisplatin alone in patients with malignant pleural mesothelioma. J Clin Oncol 21:2636–2644
5. Scherpereel A, Astoul P, Baas P et al. (2010) Guidelines of the European Respiratory Society and the European Society of Thoracic Surgeons for the management of malignant pleural mesothelioma. Eur Respir J 135(3):479–495
6. Grégoire M (2010) What's the place of immunotherapy in malignant mesothelioma treatments? Cell Adh Migr 4(1):153–161
7. Goey SH, Eggermont AM, Punt CJ, Slingerland R, Gratama JW, Oosterom R, Oskam R, Bolhuis RL, Stoter G (1995) Intrapleural administration of interleukin 2 in pleural mesothelioma: a phase I-II study. Br J Cancer 72(5):1283–1288

8. Kiselevsky MV (ed) (2012) Malignant Effusions: Pleuritis, Ascites, Pericardites. Springer, Dordrecht/New York, p 156
9. Doherty M, Leighl NB, Feld R, Bradbury PA (1999) Phase I/II study of tumor-infiltrating lymphocyte (TIL) infusion and low-dose interleukin-2 (IL-2) in patients with advanced malignant pleural mesothelioma. Ann Surg Oncol 6(3):272–278
10. Hegmans JP, Veltman JD, Lambers ME, de Vries IJ, Figdor CG, Hendriks RW, Hoogsteden HC, Lambrecht BN, Aerts JG (2010) Consolidative dendritic cell-based immunotherapy elicits cytotoxicity against malignant mesothelioma. Am J Respir Crit Care Med 181(12):1383–1390
11. Aerts J, Cornelissen R, Leest CVD et al (2017) OA13.06 autologous dendritic cells loaded with allogeneic tumor cell lysate (Pheralys®) in patients with mesothelioma: final results of a Phase I study. J Thorac Oncol 12(1):S295
12. van den Ancker W, van Luijn MM, Westers TM et al (2010) Recent advances in antigen-loaded dendritic cell-based strategies for treatment of minimal residual disease in acute myeloid leukemia. Immunotherapy 2(1):69–83
13. Cornelissen R, Lievense LA, Heuvers ME, Maat AP, Hendriks RW, Hoogsteden HC, Hegmans JP, Aerts JG (2012) Dendritic cell-based immunotherapy in mesothelioma Immunotherapy 4(10):1011–1022
14. Baas P, Buikhuisen W, Dalesio O et al (2011) A multicenter, randomized Phase III maintenance study of thalidomide (arm A) versus observation (arm B) in patients with malignant pleural mesothelioma (MPM) after induction chemotherapy. J Clin Oncol 29(Suppl): Abstract 7006
15. Jakobsen JN, Sørensen JB (2011) Review on clinical trials of targeted treatments in malignant mesothelioma. Cancer Chemother Pharmacol 68(1):1–15
16. Dubey S, Jänne PA, Krug L, Pang H, Wang X, Heinze R, Watt C, Crawford J, Kratzke R, Vokes E, Kindler HL (2010) A phase II study of sorafenib in malignant mesothelioma: results of Cancer and Leukemia Group B 30307. J Thorac Oncol 5(10):1655–1661
17. Stevenson JP, Kindler HL, Papasavvas E et al (2013) Immunological effects of the TGFbeta-blocking antibody GC1008 in malignant pleural mesothelioma patients. Oncoimmunology 2(8):e26218
18. Pardoll DM (2012) The blockade of immune checkpoints in cancer immunotherapy. Nat Rev Cancer 12(4):252–264
19. Cedres S, Ponce-Aix S, Zugazagoitia J et al (2015) Analysis of expression of programmed cell death 1 ligand 1 (PD-L1) in malignant pleural mesothelioma (MPM). PloS One 10(3):e0121071
20. Calabro L, Morra A, Fonsatti E et al (2013) Tremelimumab for patients with chemotherapy-resistant advanced malignant mesothelioma: an open-label, single-arm, phase 2 trial. Lancet Oncol 14(11):1104–1111
21. Calabro L, Morra A, Fonsatti E et al (2015) Efficacy and safety of an intensified schedule of tremelimumab for chemotherapy-resistant malignant mesothelioma: an open-label, single-arm, phase 2 study. Lancet Respir Med 3(4):301–309
22. American Association for Cancer Research [No author listed] A Potential immune therapy for mesothelioma (2015) Cancer Discov Jul; 5(7)
23. Maio M, Scherpereel A, Calabrò L, Aerts J, Perez SC, Bearz A, et al (2017) Tremelimumab as second-line or third-line treatment in relapsed malignant mesothelioma (DETERMINE): a multicentre, international, randomised, double-blind, placebo-controlled phase 2b trial. Lancet Oncol 18(9):1261–1273. https://doi.org/10.1016/S1470-2045(17)30446-1. Epub 2017 Jul 17
24. Pastan I, Hassan R (2014) Discovery of mesothelin and exploiting it as a target for immunotherapy. Cancer Res 74(11):2907–2912
25. Servais EL, Colovos C, Rodriguez L et al (2012) Mesothelin overexpression promotes mesothelioma cell invasion and MMP-9 secretion in an orthotopic mouse model and in epithelioid pleural mesothelioma patients. Clin Cancer Res 18(9):2478–2489
26. Hassan R, Schweizer C, Lu KF et al (2010) Inhibition of mesothelin-CA-125 interaction in patients with mesothelioma by the anti-mesothelin monoclonal antibody MORAb-009: Implications for cancer therapy. Lung Cancer 68(3):455–459

27. Hassan R, Cohen SJ, Phillips M et al (2010) Phase I clinical trial of the chimeric anti-mesothelin monoclonal antibody MORAb-009 in patients with mesothelin-expressing cancers. Clin Cancer Res 16(24):6132–6138
28. Hassan R, Kindler HL, Jahan T et al (2014) Phase II clinical trial of amatuximab, a chimeric antimesothelin antibody with pemetrexed and cisplatin in advanced unresectable pleural mesothelioma. Clin Cancer Res 20(23):5927–5936
29. May RJ, Dao T, Pinilla-Ibarz J et al (2007) Peptide epitopes from the Wilms' tumor 1 oncoprotein stimulate CD4+ and CD8+ T cells that recognize and kill human malignant mesothelioma tumor cells. Clin Cancer Res 13(15 Pt 1):4547–4555
30. Zolot RS, Basu S, Million RP (2013) Antibody-drug conjugates. Nat Rev Drug Discov 12(4):259–260
31. Hassan R, Lerner MR, Benbrook D et al (2002) Antitumor activity of SS(dsFv)PE38 and SS1(dsFv)PE38, recombinant antimesothelin immunotoxins against human gynecologic cancers grown in organotypic culture in vitro. Clin Cancer Res 8(11):3520–3526
32. Li Q, Verschraegen CF, Mendoza J, Hassan R (2004) Cytotoxic activity of the recombinant anti-mesothelin immunotoxin, SS1(dsFv)PE38, towards tumor cell lines established from ascites of patients with peritoneal mesotheliomas. Anticancer Res 24(3a):1327–1335
33. Hassan R, Bullock S, Premkumar A et al (2007) Phase I study of SS1P, a recombinant anti-mesothelin immunotoxin given as a bolus I.V. infusion to patients with mesothelin-expressing mesothelioma, ovarian, and pancreatic cancers. Clin Cancer Res 13(17):5144–5149
34. Kreitman RJ, Hassan R, Fitzgerald DJ, Pastan I (2009) Phase I trial of continuous infusion anti-mesothelin recombinant immunotoxin SS1P. Clin Cancer Res 15(16):5274–5279
35. Hassan R, Sharon E, Thomas A et al (2014) Phase 1 study of the antimesothelin immunotoxin SS1P in combination with pemetrexed and cisplatin for front-line therapy of pleural mesothelioma and correlation of tumor response with serum mesothelin, megakaryocyte potentiating factor, and cancer antigen 125. Cancer 120(21):3311–3319
36. Hassan R, Miller AC, Sharon E et al (2013) Major cancer regressions in mesothelioma after treatment with an anti-mesothelin immunotoxin and immune suppression. Sci Transl Med 5(208):208ra14
37. Junghans RP (2017) The challenges of solid tumors for designer CAR-T therapies: a 25-year perspective. Cancer Gene Ther 24:89–99
38. Adusumilli PS, Cherkassky L, Villena-Vargas J et al (2014) Regional delivery of mesothelin-targeted CAR T cell therapy generates potent and long-lasting CD4-dependent tumor immunity. Sci Transl Med 6(261):261ra151
39. Mayor M, Zeltsman M, McGee E (2016) Adusumilli PS A regional approach for CAR T-cell therapy for mesothelioma: from mouse models to clinical trial. Immunotherapy 8(5):491–494
40. Wang LC, Lo A, Scholler J et al (2014) Targeting fibroblast activation protein in tumor stroma with chimeric antigen receptor T cells can inhibit tumor growth and augment host immunity without severe toxicity. Cancer Immunol Res 2(2):154–166
41. Rajasagi M, Shukla SA, Fritsch EF, Keskin DB, Deluca D, Carmona E, Zhang W, Sougnez C, Cibulskis K, Sidney J et al (2014) Systematic identification of personal tumor-specific neoantigens in chronic lymphocytic leukemia. Blood 124:453–462
42. Tran E, Turcotte S, Gros A, Robbins PF, Lu YC, Dudley ME, Wunderlich JR, Somerville RP, Hogan K, Hinrichs CS et al (2014) Cancer immunotherapy based on mutation-specific CD4+ T cells in a patient with epithelial cancer. Science 344:641–645. https://doi.org/10.1126/science.1251102
43. Huang J, El-Gamil M, Dudley ME, Li YF, Rosenberg SA, Robbins PF (2004) T cells associated with tumor regression recognize frameshifted products of the CDKN2A tumor suppressor gene locus and a mutated HLA class I gene product. J Immunol 172:6057–6064
44. Hacohen N, Fritsch EF, Carter TA, Lander ES, Wu CJ (2013) Getting personal with neoantigen-based therapeutic cancer vaccines. Cancer Immunol Res 1:11–15

45. Gauvrit A, Brandler S, Sapede-Peroz C, Boisgerault N, Tangy F, Gregoire M (2008) Measles virus induces oncolysis of mesothelioma cells and allows dendritic cells to cross-prime tumor-specific CD8 response. Cancer Res 68(12):4882–4892
46. Shubina IZ, Blumenberg AG, Volkov SM, Demidov LV, Kiselevskiy MV (2007) Adoptive immunotherapy of malignant neoplasms. Vestnik RAMS 11:9–15

Index

A
Anticancer drugs, 92, 96–99
Appendiceal neoplasms, 74, 81

C
CAR-T-cells, 114, 115
Cytoreductive surgery (CRS), v, 40, 41, 43, 49–55, 57–60, 62–65, 73, 74, 76–78, 81–84, 91, 106, 112
Cytotoxicity, 55, 56, 92, 99

D
Diagnosis, v, vi, 1–15, 21, 24–29, 31, 33, 35, 36, 101, 104, 116

E
Effectors of antitumor immunity, 98
Etiology, vi, 1–15, 24, 31, 32, 65, 82, 83

H
Hyperthermia, 55
Hyperthermia, induced, 7, 44, 49, 55–57, 59, 61, 62, 65, 74, 91–99, 104, 105, 112, 114, 115

I
Immune checkpoint inhibitors, 108–109, 114, 115
Immunotherapy, v, 99, 101–117
Incidence, v, 1–15, 20, 25, 82
Intraperitoneal chemotherapy, v, 5, 7, 40, 44–49, 54–60, 62, 65, 73, 74, 77, 83–84, 91, 106

L
LAK-cells, 99, 102, 103, 117

M
Malignant mesothelioma (MM), 9–12, 20, 24–32, 101–103, 105–113
Mesothelial lesions, 19–33

N
Neoplasms, mesothelial, v, 2, 3, 6–10, 12, 14, 19–33, 35, 74, 75, 81, 84

P
Peritoneal carcinomatosis, 56, 60, 74, 84, 91
Peritoneal mesothelioma (PM), 8–15, 24, 30, 39–65, 74, 82, 84, 101
Prognosis, v, 2, 3, 6, 9, 14, 21, 24, 27, 30, 32, 33, 36, 50, 60–62, 65, 75, 77, 81–83, 101
Pseudomyxoma peritonei (PMP), v, 1–15, 33, 34, 36, 37, 39–65, 74, 75, 81, 84, 117

T
Tumor cells, 3, 4, 8, 21, 24–27, 29, 34, 35, 55, 56, 92, 95–99, 102, 103, 114, 115

© Springer Nature Switzerland AG 2019

M. V. Kiselevskiy et al. (eds.), *Malignant Mesothelioma and Pseudomyxoma*,
https://doi.org/10.1007/978-3-319-99510-6

Printed by Printforce, the Netherlands